T0292718

Nutrition of the Performance Horse

The EAAP series is published under the direction of Dr. P. Rafai

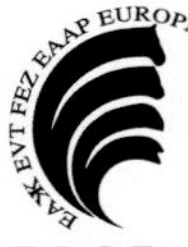

EAAP – European Association for Animal Production

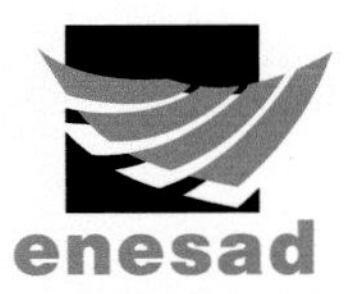

ENESAD – établissement national d'enseignement supérieur agronomique de Dijon – Nutrition and digestive health of herbivores

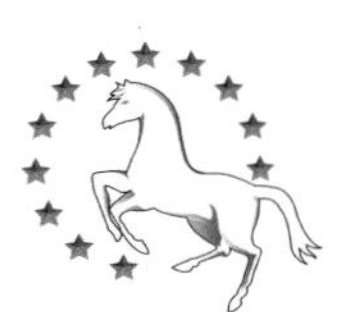

European Workshop on Equine Nutrition

The European Association for Animal Production wishes to express its appreciation to the *Ministero per le Politiche Agricole e Forestali* and the *Associazione Italiana Allevatori* for their valuable support of its activities

Nutrition of the Performance Horse

Which system in Europe for evaluating the nutritional requirements?

EAAP publication No. 111

Editors:

V. Julliand and W. Martin-Rosset

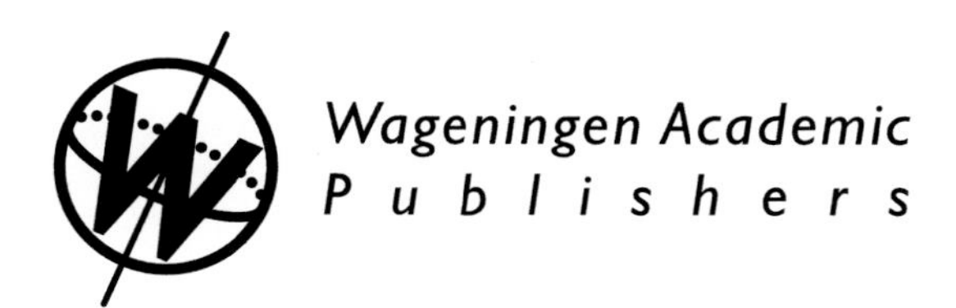

CIP-data Koninklijke Bibliotheek, Den Haag

ISBN 907699837X paperback
ISSN 0071-2477

Subject headings:
Equine
Animal nutrition
Nutritional systems

First published, 2004

Wageningen Academic Publishers
The Netherlands, 2004

Foreword

The Horse Commission of the European Association for Animal Production (EAAP) uses to perform, in the scope of annual meetings of EAAP, scientific sessions devoted either to a disciplinary area to investigate new concepts, methodologies and tools, or to a multidisciplinary approach to answer multifactorial questions arising from Equine industry.

More recently different working groups have been set up under the umbrella of the Horse Commission to examine thoroughly the scientific thought and to contribute to the settlement of European network for research and the harmonisation of methodology and tools to be implemented in Horse production. These working groups are developing activities all the year long between two subsequent annual meetings of EAAP. Workshops are performed by these working groups. They are carried out in different European Countries which volunteer to organise them. Projects of R & D are sometimes set up and implemented by several European Countries. The papers prepared and presented during these workshops are published either as internal report or increasingly as scientific issue in Livestock Production Science or in Special EAAP series.

Thanks to the initiative of the research group "UPR Nutrition des Herbivores" of ENESAD (Etablissement National Enseignement Supérieur Agronomique de Dijon) leaded by Veronique Julliand, a European Workshop on Equine Nutrition was organised in 2002 in France. This workshop was performed in Dijon on January 15-17th and it was focused on the topic of "Nutritional Systems for Equines".

In 2002, the recommended allowances for Equines are evaluated in the different European Countries using either the American Systems of NRC, or the French systems of INRA with or without adaptation to encounter the local background . The allowances are evaluated either using Digestible Energy (DE) and Crude Protein (CP) of NRC systems or using Net Energy (NE) and Horse Digestible Crude Protein (HDCP so called MADC in French) of INRA systems. The allowances of mineral and vitamins are evaluated using the same scientific bases whatever the main countries due to the lack of knowledge.

It is of great concern to clarify the situation and to promote the harmonisation of the nutritional systems to be used in Europe to make easier the commercial exchanges in the European horse industry - namely the feed industry. The European group of research on Equine Nutrition should be partner to carry out the studies in the area as it is requested by the European Commission, namely in the scope of the Framework Programme of R & D designed to promote a European network for research.

Several attempts were initiated in the nineties to promote a brain storming in the area of nutritional systems under the umbrella of the Horse Commission.

In 1993, a European Workshop was performed in Reyjkavik by Island and the proceedings were published in a special issue of Livestock Production Science (Livest. Prod. Sci., 1994, 40) edited by O. Gudmunsson, who leaded the organisation of the workshop.

In 1996, a full session devoted to the Nutritional System was performed by W. Martin-Rosset and D. Austbø in the scope of the scientific program carried out by the Horse Commission during the 47th Annual EAAP Meeting held in Lillehammer (Norway)

The new workshop performed in Dijon in 2002, is promoting again the process. It should be continued every two years and performed by a European Country which volunteers under the umbrella of the Horse Commission of EAAP. As a result this proceedings and the next following ones will be published as a special issue of a new scientific series of EAAP,. similarly to the proceedings of Energy or/and Protein Metabolism Meetings which are carried out by the Commission on Nutrition.

This kind of publication should improve the dissemination of consistent scientific knowledge to help the end users to match the new challenge that Equine industry has to face with the booming of horse production and utilisation at the early stage of 21st century. It should promote a European network for research in Equine nutrition as well.

W. Martin-Rosset
President of Horse Commission

Contents

Representations of equestrian structures managers on horse nutrition

Franck Rémond

UPR Nutrition des Herbivores, Département des sciences et techniques agronomiques, ENESAD, Dijon, France

1. Problematic

Few studies were interested in knowledge, well known or only used, by horses "stockbreeders", and have confronted them with the theoretical knowledge diffused by the scientists and other actors of the horse industry.

The meaning of these theoretical knowledge for the people in charge of feeding (which one will be called CA in this article) is not known, and we ignore if the message emitted by scientists are well-understood by this CA. One can then ask the following question: does there exist common meaning to the various actors of the horse industry? The use of common meaning by the various partners is however particularly significant in the processes of communication: "*to understand ourselves, therefore to establish a relation of communication, one implements same meaning as the neighbours, so that they can recognize them* " (Lamizet and Silem, 1997, p515).

A pre study allow to put forth assumptions on the differences of opinion between the professional practices of the CA, based on some knowledge and the messages transmitted by the scientists: this investigation (Rémond, 2000) revealed that on the 13 surveyed people, none truly used the systems created by the scientists to describe the food (systems UFC and MADC). However 3 people had spoken about the energy value of food, which approaches UFC concept. The surveyed people more easily approached the protein rate of food. Or they stated that they don't know its characteristics, because they were rather using their practical knowledge to manage the feeding. The theoretical knowledge, resulting from scientific research, would thus not be adopted by CA, which would use their experiment, their practical knowledge to carry out the tasks which income to them.

A problematic, depending of the communication and information sciences, and talking about the equine nutrition would be thus to develop, with for objective improving this communication (or popularization) and installing a beginning of synergy between the various actors of the horse industry. Indeed processes of efficient information and comprehension must be used to ensure correct use, by these CA, of the scientific research carried out in this field.

The study presented here aimed to study the context in which information currently arrives, i.e. the meaning allotted to the feeding by CA of equestrian structures, their representations on this topic. "*the social representation is a process of perceptive and mental elaboration of the reality which transforms the social objects (people, contexts, situations) into symbolic categories (values, beliefs, ideologies) and confers to them a cognitive statute making it possible to apprehend the aspects of the ordinary life by a realignment of our own behaviour inside the social interactions* " (Fischer, 1987). It would be thus more simply a mental activity through which one makes present at the spirit, by an image, an absent object or event.

2. Methodology

To study the representations of the CA, depending of the systems of values of the individuals, and producing the meaning of the practices and knowledges of the CA, (Lamizet and Silem, 1997 p 478), the technique selected was the realization of semi-directive interviews in an heterogeneous sample of CA. The study is indeed in an exploratory and qualitative process. Having only few information at the beginning, "*the significant one is not to know if one measures well what one is supposed to measure, but only to recognize what one discovers* " (Grawitz, 1996). The constitution of the sample thus consisted in diversifying to the maximum the people questioned in order to not forget any significant situation.

In the same way, the interview questionnaire set up for these investigations, only indicates to the investigator the topics to be approached and aims to leave the interviewed structure himself its mind. Each interview is thus carried out differently, and one of the difficulties for the investigator is to remain rigorous in its research of information. Moreover it is significant to note that the investigator must adopt an interview method allowing the interviewed explaining his personal point of view, this in order to find the reality seen by this last.

The method of analysis used approaches the analysis of contents. The material collected at the time of the investigations was retranscribed, then compared and classified in relevant categories. These categories, formed according to the initial assumptions of the study, are refined according to the investigations carried out, but are also initially used to improve the interview questionnaire. When the new investigations do not allow any more increase in the categories accuracy, the sample can be regarded as sufficient.

3. Results and discussion

For this study, 11 investigations were carried out in structures of leisures, teaching, competition, and working in CSO, Dressage, 3 days events, Endurance, and hunting.

The speeches of surveyed were, like this was higher explained, gathered into categories of answers and a synthesis of the whole answers allow to find systems of values more or less significant according to the type of structure.

A strong and commune concept of the various systems of representations were found for the whole surveyed people (whatever is the sports activity, the level of competition and the size of the structure). It is the concept of body score of the horse. This concept would guide them in their practices and corresponds to the aim they had as CA. This concept, which remains however fuzzy enough for CA, is the main term associated with the feeding, the image which is associated there. A joint definition could be "*a horse with a good musculature and without fat* ", but other elements can integrated in this definition, and this differently according to each CA. The evaluation of this body score condition is done primarily visually "*it is necessary to have a good glance* ". The body score evaluation of the horse allows them to evaluate their own work and also the one of the others. CA thus seek to adapt their practices to the body score of the horse.

The meaning allotted to the feeding can be then based on more or less significant values according to the types of CA, but always in relation the ones with the others. The representations are based on complex systems of values which cannot be really studied separately. Among these values we find:

- Functionality of the feeding:

The importance of a practical feeding (easy to make, not asking too much time and storage capacity), "*which should not be a drudgery* " (structure I), was especially stressed by the exclusive factory feedstuff users. Thus for certain CA, the feeding should not require too much personal implication and could even be managed by the food manufacturer. But the exclusive factory feedstuff users are not the only ones to have this functional image of the feeding. One finds this concern on the level of the issue of rations, which is allotted to another person of the structure, by CA using only traditional cereals.

- The financial aspect.

The structures using traditional cereals in particular justified this decision by the fact that the cereals were less expensive than factory feedstuffs. The financial value thus takes for them the advantage on the value functionality.

- The good being of the horse.

The feeding would be for these people (primarily CA using traditional cereals) something making it possible to bring pleasure to the horse.

To have an image of reality not asking too much cognitive effort, the individuals have recourse to a process called schematization of reality. This one consists in simplifying reality for better controlling it. This process were materialized in the investigations by the fact that CA used enormously their practical knowledge and very little their theoretical knowledge. The estimation of the rations is done thus, for the whole of the surveyed people, thanks to the experiment which they acquired in this field by observing the results on the horse. It is necessary, according to them, to observe and especially know their horses.

One of the questions of the investigations was interested particularly in the method of estimation of the rations and was formulated in the following way:
How is it necessary to make, according to you, the evaluation of the horse ration ?
Various types of information are arisen from the analysis of this question:

- The role and the responsibility of the CA in the estimation of the rations:

Certain CA leave the feed manufacturer provide this function in their structure. This can let think that the calculation (or the estimation) of the rations does not make party of their work, or at least that they do not consider themselves like the most qualified in the field, and that a help is sometimes necessary for them (this with an aim of improving the effectiveness of the feeding or to limit the working time on this activity).

Other CA do not call upon the manufacturer but use the impersonal information provided by the manufacturers (labels) to estimate the rations. It is then surprising to see that some of these CA do not control this information, since they do not know which quantity of food they give to their horses (the volume and the weight contained in can of distribution is not known).
Finally, other CA do not call upon any external person to carry out this operation.

- Rationing technique of CA:

The adaptation of the ration to the horse would be done according to the observations made on their horses and according to the reaction of this one to the ration. This mean that they use the practical knowledge that they acquired with the experiment learnt in the reality. One finds speeches like
"*if it is wrong (the ration), one immediately sees it... with the body score of the horse, with his appetite, with his behaviour: If he pulls the barouche as well the evening as the morning, it is that it is good* ".

"It is necessary to be accustomed to seeing the horses, it is necessary to know them and to know what have changed and to know changing its ration "
One of the main signs to take into account in the estimation of the ration to come would be in fact the result of the preceding ration on the horse (body score, behaviour at work). However it should not be said that it is the only sign since many of other elements like anticipation on coming work or health in particular, were also underlined.

The theoretical knowledge would be not used by CA. Some of them own this theoretical knowledge and are able to explain the functioning of systems UFC and MADC but state not to use these systems because they would not correspond to their daily concerns. One finds citation like:
"*one could calculate the ration within a gram with a calculator, but it should be remembered that the distribution is done by can, that it is vague, therefore finally one does it with the feeling... in fact the observation is better*".
"*for a horse, it should be done with the eye, for the bovine one it was necessary to calculate the rations, but the horse it is not similar, one does not seek a GMQ (daily average profit of weight) or anything. That is not the similar thing, that can change from a day to the following day* "
"*here there are no time (to make calculations), one tests, one sees whether it is good, and then one makes*"

It is also interesting to note that CA which are able to describe in a more pointed way the techniques of rationing, declared in fact to be interested personally in the feeding of the horse but which they thought that it was not profitable to reason so finely:
"*there are calculations when a ration is made, but the most significant one is the eye... to feed finely is not profitable and me I do it by passion*".

The process of representation of CA thus passes by a schematization of the reality in which are mainly retained the observations made in the practical reality and the practices to be adopted according to those ones. The systems of assessment needs and energy and protein contributions to horse are not used; if the result is good on the body score of the horse, it is that the feed is of good quality. Moreover for certain people, the theoretical concerns would not be a part of their job but a part of the manufacturers job.

CA thus use enormously their practical knowledge and limit the relevance of the theoretical knowledge in their daily practices. This confirms the results of Rémond (2000): the food reality seen by CA do not relate the criteria used by the zootechnicians to describe this same activity and the messages diffused by the latter one must thus be based on values like the functionality of the feeding, the financial aspect, the good being of the horse and especially the body score of the horse to find a good meaning for CA.

References

Fischer, G.N., 1987. Les concepts fondamentaux de la psychologie sociale. *Bordas, Paris,* 206 p.

Grawitz, M., 1996. Livre 3; les techniques au service des sciences sociales. In: *Précis de méthodes des sciences sociales 10ième édition, Grawitz, M (1996). Editions Dalloz, Paris. 860 p.* pp 443-789.

Lamizet B. and Silem, A., 1997. Dictionnaire encyclopédique des sciences de l'information et de la communication. Ellipses, édition marketing SA, Paris, 590 p

Remond F., 2001. Analyse des représentations des professionnels chargés d'alimentation dans les structures équestres. *Mémoire de DEA Lettres, Humanités, Civilisations, option information, communication. Université de Bourgogne.* 90p.

Remond, F., 2000. Implication de l'alimentation dans les pathologies du cheval: enquêtes auprès de professionnels équins. *Mémoire d'ingénieur, ENESAD.* 38 p.

European systems used for evaluating the energy requirements of performance horses

Digestible energy requirements of horses for maintenance and work

Gary D. Potter

Equine Sciences, Texas A&M University, USA

1. Energy partitioning

The following scheme of partitioning the use of dietary energy applies to horses in the same manner as all species of animals:

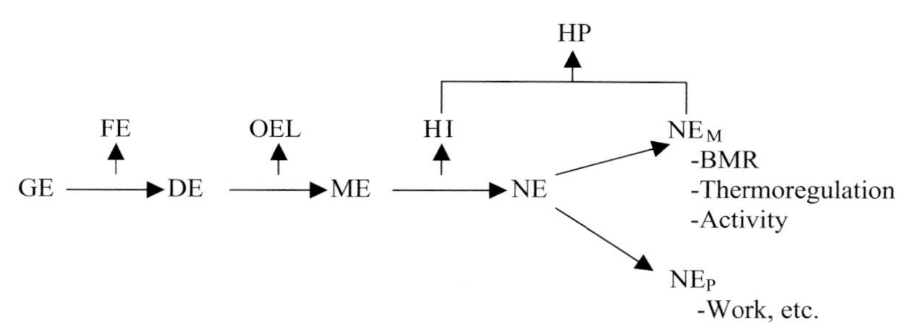

where,

GE = total combustible energy in the diet
FE = energy lost in feces
OEL = energy lost in urine and gasses escaping from the digestive tract
HI = energy lost as heat due to the digestive process
HP = energy lost as the total heat production of the animal
DE = energy absorbed
ME = metabolizable energy
NE = net energy available for maintenance and productive use
NE_M = net energy required for maintenance
NE_P = net energy available for productive use

In deciding how to define the energy requirements of horses, one must decide what expression to use, ie. GE, DE, ME, NE, NE_M or NE_P. GE is a rather useless expression to define energy requirements of animals, because the GE concentration in all feedstuffs of comparable chemical composition is very similar. However, the digestibility of that energy is highly variable depending on the proportion of such constituents as structural carbohydrates vs. nonstructural carbohydrates, ether extract and protein. Thus, one major refinement in the definition of energy requirements relative to the energy in feedstuffs is to define the requirements in terms of DE. The NRC (1989) chose to define energy requirements of horses in terms of DE. As will be shown later, the level of refinement when defining energy requirements in terms of DE is limited because several environmental factors and factors in the metabolic process can affect the DE requirement of horses in a given situation.

It is commonly held that the BMR of land mammals is approximately 70 kcal/kgBW$^{.75}$. There is little reason to assume that the BMR of horses is different than that of other animals. Also, for many animals, it is commonly held that when energy losses in urine, gasses escaping from the digestive tract and heat are accounted, the DE requirement is approximately twice the BMR, or

140 kcal/kgBW$^{.75}$. Early versions of the NRC requirements for maintenance of horses held close to that relationship (NRC, 1973).

2. Factors affecting theDErequirement for maintenance of the exercising horse

2.1 Environmental temperature

The horse has a very efficient mechanism for thermoregulation, and thus, within the zone of thermal neutrality, the variation in NE_M for thermoregulation in horses is negligible. However, when horses are maintained in environments where the ambient temperature is below approximately 15°C or above approximately 30°C, the NE_M is increased, and thus, NE, ME andDErequirements are increased. However, the exact lower and upper temperatures that define the zone of thermal neutrality in the horse are not clear. NRC (1989) concluded that there were insufficient data in the literature to account for thermal challenge, and no adjustment in the DE for maintenance was made for thermoregulation when horses are maintained in an environment outside the zone of thermal neutrality. However, Potter et al. (1990) demonstrated that horses exercised at the same workload in temperate weather (17°C; 60% relative humidity) vs. hot weather (32°C; 45% relative humidity) required different amounts of DE to maintain body weight and composition (Table 1). From this work and other, it is clear that environmental conditions affect the energy requirements of athletic horses. Thus, more research is needed to determine regression coefficients that could be used in a model to predict energy requirements when horses are maintained outside the zone of thermal neutrality, thus, moving to more of a NE description of energy requirements.

Table 1. Digestible energy requirements of exercising horses for work and maintenance in different seasons of the year and fed a conventional diet (Potter et al., 1990).

	Temperate weather	Hot weather
Body wt., kg	489	477
DE, Mcal/d	18.5	19.2*
DE, work	3.9	3.8
DE, main.	14.7	15.4*

*P<.05

2.2 Composition of the body

In addition to environmental conditions, the composition of the horse's body affects the efficiency of thermal regulation. When horses are too lean, there may be excessive heat lost from the body in cold weather, thus increasing the energy requirements. When NRC (1989) was published, there were insufficient data available to make such adjustments. Later, Potter et al. (1990) found that excessive body fat content increased the DE requirement in horses exercising in temperate or hot weather (Table 2). Clearly horses with excessive body fat content require more energy to dissipate heat than horses in leaner condition, particularly in temperate and hot weather. One could speculate from these data that horses in too lean condition would similarly need extra energy for thermoregulation in colder weather. Thus, more research is needed to develop regression equations to predict the influence of body composition on energy requirements-again, moving more toward a NE expression of energy requirements.

Table 2. Digestible energy requirements for work and maintenance in exercising horses maintained in different body conditions and fed a conventional diet (Potter et al., 1990).

	Moderate condition	Fleshy condition
Body wt., kg	465	503
DE, Mcal/d	15.4	22.3*
DE, work	3.7	4.0
DE, main.	11.7	18.4*

*P<.05

2.3 Composition of the diet

Energy lost as heat from the work of digestion can vary widely in horses depending on the composition of the diet. Diets that result in comparatively more fermentive digestion in the large intestine vs. mammalian enzymatic digestion in the small intestine will be more thermogenic. Kane et al. (1979) and Scott et al. (1993) found that adding fat to the equine diet increases the useable energy of the diet without significantly increasing heat production. Potter et al. (1990) found that when exercising horses were worked at constant workload, substituting fat for some of the nonstructural carbohydrates in the diet resulted in significant reduction of the DE required for maintenance of body weight and condition (Table 3).

Table 3. Digestible energy requirements for work and maintenance in exercising horses fed a conventional diet or fat-supplemented diet, and maintained in moderate condition (Potter et al., 1990).

	Conventional diet	Fat-supplemented diet
Body wt., kg	465	463
DE, Mcal/d	15.4	12.8*
DE, work	3.7	3.7
DE, main.	11.7	9.1*

*P<.05

2.4 Interactive effects

Data in Tables 1-3 clearly indicate that the DE requirements of exercising horses in all conditions cannot be predicted accurately by simple extrapolation from body weight and workload. Adjustments must be made for environmental conditions, composition of the body and composition of the diet. Table 4 shows a comparative index reflecting how each of the above conditions affects the DE required for maintenance of horses doing similar amounts of work. For comparative purposes, the DE required for maintenance of horses in moderate flesh, fed a conventional diet and maintained in moderate condition is set at 100, and the other requirements are indexed to that level. It is clear that all three factors affect the DE requirements of horses, thus regressions to predict the effects of all three factors are needed to refine the prediction of the actual energy requirements of exercising horses maintained under different conditions and fed different diets.

Table 4. Index of DE requirements of exercising horses under different conditions (Potter et al., 1990).

Moderate Body Condition	Index
Conventional diet, temperate weather	100
Conventional diet, hot weather	115
Fat-suppl. diet, temperate weather	75
Fat-suppl. diet, hot weather	92
Fleshy Body Condition	
Conventional diet, temperate weather	155
Conventional diet, hot weather	161
Fat-suppl. diet, temperate weather	139
Fat-suppl. diet, hot weather	154

3. Defining theDErequirements for work

The NRC (1989) focused on two methods of calculating the DE requirements for working horses. The regression equation of Anderson et al. (1983) predicts the total DE requirement for maintenance and work of horses doing intense exercise in a range up to approximately 4,000 kg•km of work daily. That regression accounts for body weight, the weight carried by the horse and the distance traveled, and is reasonably predictive of the total DE requirement of exercising horses. However, the equation tends to overestimate slightly the actual DE requirements of horses galloping on a track because data used to develop the regression were obtained from horses working on a treadmill. Even though fans were used to simulate wind conditions on the track, it appears that horses galloping on a track may have a more efficient mechanism of dissipating heat than horses worked on a treadmill, thus a lower NE_M. The equation of Pagan and Hintz (1986) estimates the DE above maintenance as a function of speed. However, the equation is of limited use in horses working at speeds in excess of 350 m/min, because it underestimates the actual requirements of horses working at faster speeds.

Table 5 shows a direct comparison of the actual DE required by 5 exercising horses with requirements predicted by the two equations referenced by NRC (1989). In this experiment, 5 mature geldings were slow-galloped varying distances on a dirt track and fed to maintain constant body weight. Energy digestibility was determined after working at each distance for two weeks. The actual daily DE required for work and maintenance of constant body weight was compared to estimated requirements using the equations of Anderson et al. (1983) and Pagan and Hintz (1986). The equation of Anderson et al. (1983) overestimated the actual DE requirements by an average

Table 5. Comparative daily DE requirements of five exercising horses

Weight kg	Distance km	Workload kg·km (times 10^{-3})	Speed m/min	Time hr	Actual mcal/d	Anderson mcal/d	Pagan mcal/d
480	0	N/A	N/A	N/A	16.8	16.1	15.8
547	2.8	1.5	440	0.11	21.6	22.6	18.1
548	5.6	3.0	440	0.21	23.7	26.9	21.5
548	11.2	6.0	440	0.42	26.6	29.0	24.1

of 9%, again likely due to the NE_M for thermoregulation being increased when horses were worked in the treadmill. The equation of Pagan and Hintz (1986) underestimated the DE requirements by an average of 13%, likely due to the inapplicability of the equation to exercise conducted at faster speeds. That equation was developed from experiments using indirect calorimetry, which is dependent on accurate measurement of oxygen consumption at varying speeds. Apparently the rate of oxygen consumption measured in those studies is not applicable for indirect calorimetric measures of energy expenditure when horses work at speeds higher than 350 m/min.

As is true for determining energy requirements for maintenance, accurate accounting of the NE_P and all the factors affecting the NE_M, the HI and OEL in the working horse are needed to prescribe energy requirements in some term more refined than DE. At the publication of NRC (1989) there were insufficient data in the literature for such accounting. Thus, energy requirements for the working horse were given in terms of DE. There are some more data available in 2001, but considerable research is still needed to refine energy requirements for working horses to NE or even NE_M and NE_P.

References

Anderson, C.E., Potter, G.D., Kreider, J.L. and Courtney, C.C., 1983. Digestible energy requirements for exercising horses. J. Anim.Sci. 56: 91

Kane, E., Baker, J.P. and Bull, L.S., 1979. Utilization of a corn oil supplemented diet by the pony. J. Anim. Sci. 48: 1379.

National Research Council, 1989. Nutrient Requirements of Horses. 5th rev. ed. Washington, D.C.: National Academy Press.

National Research Council, 1973. Nutrient Requirements of Horses. 4th rev. ed. Washington, D.C.: National Academy Press.

Pagan, J.D. and Hintz,. H.F., 1986. Equine energetics II. Energy expenditure in hoses during submaximal exercise. J. Anim. Sci. 63: 822.

Potter, G.D., Webb, S.P., Evans, J.W. and Webb, G.W., 1990. Digestible energy requirements for work and maintenance of horses fed conventional and fat-supplemented diets. J. Equine Vet. Sci. 10(3): 214.

Scott, B.D., Potter, G.D., Greene, L.W., Vogelsang, M.M. and Anderson, J.G., 1993. Efficacy of a fat-supplemented diet to reduce thermal stress in exercising Thoroughbred horses. Proc. 13th Equine Nutr. Phys. Symp. p. 66.

The German system (digestible energy)

Ellen Kienzle

Institute for Animal Physiology, Physiological Chemistry and Animal Nutrition, Ludwig-Maximilians-University Munich, Germany

Energy evaluation of feed and the determination of energy requirements are two ways of looking at one issue (figure 1), i.e. the transformation of the gross energy (heat of combustion) in the feed into energy used for a certain performance (including maintenance) of the animal. The transformation of the energy occurs in several steps, beginning with the losses of energy during digestion and ending with the heat losses during performance. Depending on the system of energy evaluation these steps are either covered by the system used for energy evaluation of the feed or by the requirement figures. In the latter case the requirement figures would include average estimates of transformation. For instance, a requirement figure for lactation expressed in metabolisable energy (ME) includes an estimate for average transformation of ME into net energy (NE) for milk production, which is usually a coefficient of utilisation of about 0.6 to 0.75. If the transformation is covered by the system of energy evaluation the transformation of the energy in different feeds is included into the unit. For instance, a net energy system for milk production requires knowledge on the transformation of ME into NE for milk production for most feed used for the species! The coefficient of utilisation is then adapted for each individual feed. Finally, any system of energy evaluation requires predictive equations for feed using chemical analyses and/or in vitro-tests to make it useful in practice.

It is relatively easy to acquire the necessary knowledge at either end of the bars in figure 1. From the point of view of feed evaluation the easiest system would be to determine heat of combustion

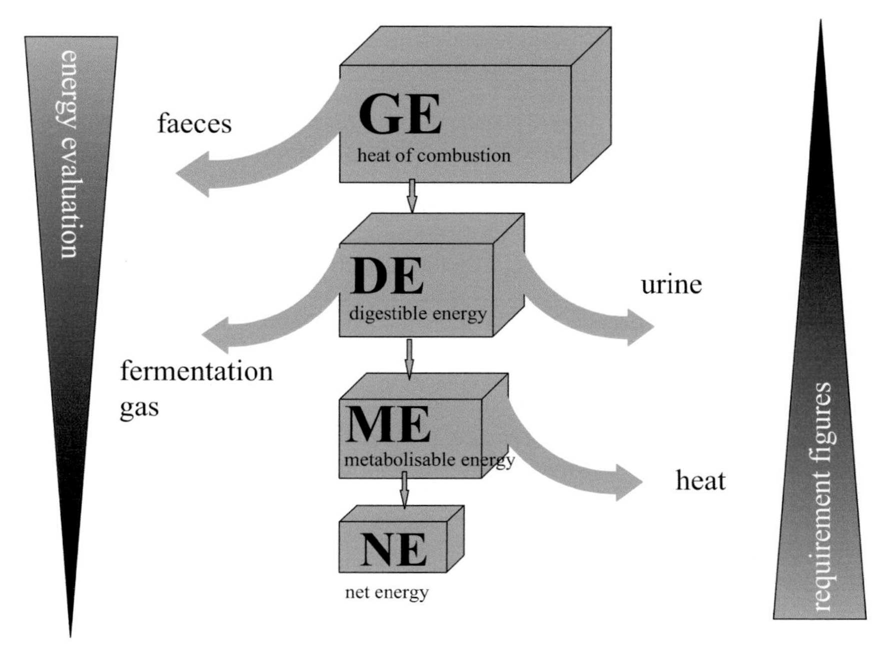

Figure 1. Two ways of looking at bioavailability of energy.

(GE) in the feed. From the point of view of requirement figures NE (or sometimes ME) is the method of choice. NE for lactation, for instance, is simply the heat of combustion in the milk. To make the system work, however, both views need to be considered. In case of a GE-system there should be very little variation in all steps of transformation in relation to feed composition, otherwise it would become very inaccurate. No GE-system is in use for any domestic species. Such a system might work in a nutritionally highly specialised animal, which eats a diet with very little variation in digestibility such as nectar eating birds. A NE-system on the other hand requires detailed knowledge on each of the steps of transformation, i.e. on intestinal and intermediary metabolism of many different feeds. Especially the knowledge on intestinal metabolism is species specific and cannot be taken from other species. Another point is that the utilisation of ME is different for different purposes (see Kleiber, 1961). For maintenance and lactation the utilisation coefficient is supposed to be somewhere around 0.6 to 0.75 for most species, for tissue accretion during growth the range is even larger (0.35 to 0.75, depending on the relation of protein and fat in the accretion), and for physical activity it is only about 0.25-0.30 (see Kamphues et al., 1999). The latter coefficient depends on several factors linked to the animal such as speed, gait and fitness. The modification of the utilisation coefficient by the feed composition is again different for different types of performance. That means that any net energy system can only be valid for one type of performance such as lactation or growth or maintenance. In theory for an animal which is not in a maintenance stage two systems would be required: net energy for maintenance and net energy for performance. Of course this is not practical. Therefore in net energy systems maintenance requirements are often expressed in net energy units for performance. This works best if i) the utilisation coefficients for maintenance and performance are similar, ii) the utilisation coefficient does not depend on individual animal related factors, and ii) maintenance requirements are much lower than requirements for performance. All three preconditions are fulfilled in dairy cows. This is probably an important reason why net energy systems are in use for dairy cows all over the world.

In horses there is a large number of digestibility studies including many types of feed. However, feed stuff interact with each other and therefore an additive system of DE values is only valid within certain limits (Zeyner and Kienzle, 2002). For instance in a ration with large percentages of straw the energy digestibility of straw may be anywhere between 30 and 50% depending on the other feed stuff in the ration (Schmidt, 1980; Lindemann, 1982; Kienzle et al., 2002). Other interactions have been observed for high fat and sometimes for high starch diets (Hollands and Cuddeford, 1992; Zeyner, 1995; Zeyner, 2001). Figures for DE requirements are mostly determined by feeding a known amount of DE while recording body weight or keeping it constant, and in part transformed from ME-values obtained by indirect calorimetry. This is not very satisfactory. In addition in a species which relies heavily on intestinal fermentation for its energy requirements the loss of fermentation gases is an important point which is not covered by a DE system. Preconditions for a ME-system would be i) quantitative knowledge on energy losses by urine in relation to protein intake, ii) quantititive knowledge on the percentage of the feed which is digested by fermentation, and iii) quantitative knowledge on the gas production during fermentation.

Some knowledge on urine energy excretion exists (Pagan and Hintz, 1986) suggesting that the horse is similar to the ruminants in that respect. It would be relatively simple to improve our knowledge by balance studies measuring urinary energy losses in relation to protein intake. The second precondition for a ME-system, the knowledge on the percentage of feed which is digested by microbial fermentation is more difficult to obtain. Starch plays an important role in horse diets. The capacity of the horse to digest starch by amylase is not as high as in pigs, but rather comparable to ruminants' small intestinal amylase activity (Kienzle et al., 1994). To measure the percentage of starch digested by amylase and maltase and absorbed as glucose small intestinal starch digestibility has been used as a rough indicator. To obtain data on this parameter small intestinal cannulas are required. Post mortem spot sampling does not give accurate results (Wilke, 1992). Depending on source, meal size and processing small intestinal starch digestibility of cereals ranges from 20 to 90% (Potter et al., 1992a; Kienzle, 1994; Meyer et al., 1995). Results are sometimes contradictory. In addition interactions between concentrate and hay have been demonstrated for small intestinal starch digestibility (Meyer et al., 1993; Meyer et al., 1995). Small intestinal protein digestibility appears to vary in a similar way (Potter et al., 1992b; Wilke, 1992). So far our knowledge on the reasons for the variation is limited. This precludes scientific justification of a ME-system in the horse. It also precludes the development of predictive equations from chemical analyses and/or in vitro-tests of feed, which is a very important point for practical application of a system. Hindgut fermentation, though in principle similar to rumen fermentation, is different between hindgut fermenters, even if they eat a comparable diet. Experiences with hindgut fermenters in zoos show that there are remarkable differences between species, for instance between elephants and horses (Loehlein, 1999). Therefore species specific quantitative data for hind gut fermentation of horses would be required for a ME-system. From qualitative research it is known that hindgut fermentation in the horse is modified by the amounts of starch and protein which flow into the hindgut (Meyer et al., 1982; Zentek et al., 1992; Kollarczik et al., 1992; Fombelle et al., 2000; McLean et al., 2000). Consequently without direct or indirect knowledge on small intestinal digestibility knowledge on hindgut fermentation cannot be applied. For all these reasons systems higher than DE would require very close limitations on the type of feed and ration (including a defined type of starch in the ration) to which they could be applied.

For a NE-system even more knowledge is required. The transformation of ME into the various net energy types for performance in the horse has not been thoroughly investigated. Even though the intermediary metabolism of all mammals is biochemically similar in principle, however, there are species differences. The horse is phylogenetically older than the ruminant or the pig. Therefore it appears reasonable to check whether values from other species are applicable to the horse before using them. In the past scientists in both parts of Germany arrived independently at the conclusion that there are not enough data to support systems higher than DE in the horse. Interestingly the Eastern Germans - in the tradition of Oskar Kellner - tried to develop a net energy system, which was dropped for lack of data supporting it.

In nutrition consultation practice there are usually two stumbling blocks for the application of any system: i) prediction of energy in feed from chemical analysis or in-vitro-tests and ii) the energy requirements of the individual animal.

For DE numerous predictive equations have been derived which are valid within certain limits of feed and ration types (Schulze, 1987; Zeyner et al., 1992; Zeyner, 1995; Fehrle, 1999; Zeyner und Kienzle, 2001 and 2002). A very important point in this context is that any equation is only valid in context with certain types of rations, otherwise interactions between feed stuffs can lead to considerable errors. An equation to predict DE from proximate nutrients which covers a large number of practical rations has been suggested by Zeyner and Kienzle (2001 and 2002) for feeds and rations with less than 35% crude fibre and less than 8% crude fat in dry matter:
DE [MJ/kg dm] = -3.66 + 0.211 protein + 0.421 fat + 0.015 fibre + 0.189 N-free extract [crude nutrients in % dm; $r = 0.992^{***}$, $\pm s = 1.236$)
An in vitro-tests to predict DE was developed by Lowman et al. (1999).

To predict individual energy requirements of horses is much more difficult. An equation using metabolic body weight gives only a very rough estimate. What exponent should be used to calculate metabolic body weight in the horse? Pagan and Hintz (1986) in a study with 4 horses of different body weight (breeds unspecified) questioned the mass exponent of 0.75 for intra-specific use in horses and suggested a linear equation with an intercept. From practical experience breed differences are known, such as a lower energy requirements for most ponies. Therefore it is not possible to use data for ponies at one end and for warmblooded or thoroughbred horses at the other end, and calculate the mass exponent which gives the best fit. The interactions between breed and body size would almost certainly lead to an overestimation of the exponent. Data from Shire horses who are supposed to be more like ponies than like light riding horses, and warmblooded horses would probably lead to an underestimation of the exponent. Similar experiences have been made in dogs (Kienzle and Rainbird, 1991). Training stage (muscle mass), body condition and exercise play an important role for individual energy requirements. Husbandry is another factor we know mostly from practical experience. A horse kept outdoors with a shelter needs more energy than a horse kept indoors in a box, especially in a cold environment. There are breed differences in cold tolerance partly due to length of hair, even in adapted horses. Does an Iceland horse need less extra energy in a cold environment than a warmblooded horse? And finally there are differences, which cannot be explained by obvious parameters. Horses from the same breed under the same conditions, even trained by the same person, may have a very different energy requirement. For instance, Zmija (1991) showed a range of energy intake between race horses in full training from 85-141 MJ DE in trotters and from 78-176 MJ DE in galoppers. Temperament and excitement during training is supposed to play a role. Even under standardised experimental conditions individual differences may be high. Stillions and Nelson (1972) measured energy requirements to maintain body weight in six mature quarter horse geldings on the same diet. The horses were allowed only enough exercise to prevent clinical signs of lack of exercise such as anorexia and edema of the legs. The horse with the highest requirements ate 81 MJ DE to maintain a body weight of 438 kg, the horse with the lowest energy intake maintained his body weight of 426 kg eating only 52 MJ DE.

In nutrition consultation practice the best way to deal with the problem of the individual energy requirement is a thorough nutritional history, calculation of the energy in the ration eaten so far, and body condition assessment. If body condition is ideal and the nutritional history is reliable the energy intake in the ration eaten so far is very close to the energy requirement of the horse. If body condition is too fat or too lean the ration eaten so far is a good starting point for changes.

References

Fehrle, S., 1999. Untersuchungen zur Verdaulichkeit von Mischfutter beim Pferd in Abhängigkeit von der Rauhfutteraufnahme. München, Tierärztliche Fakultät der Ludwig-Maximilians-Universität, Dissertation.

Fombelle de, A., Medina, B., Drogoul, C., Jacotot, E., Reibel, C., Julliand, V. and Fombelle de, A., 2000. Variable proportions of cereals in the diet; effects on digestive function (Distribuer une proportion varible de cereales dans la ration: conse-quences sur le fonctionnement du systeme digestif). 26e Journee de la recherche equine, 1 mars 2000, 33-43.

Hollands, T. and Cuddeford, D., 1992. Einfluß einer Sojaölsupplementation auf die Nährstoffverdaulichkeit einer Rauhfutter-Kraftfutter-Ration (40:60) bei Pferden (Effect of supplementary soya oil on the digestibility of nutrients contained in a 40:60 roughage concentrate diet fed to horses). Pferdeheilkunde, Sonderausgabe, 128-132.

Kamphues, J., Schneider, D. and Leibetseder, J., 1999. Supplemente zu Vorlesungen und Übungen in der Tierernährung. Verlag M. & H. Schaper, Alfeld-Hannover.

Kienzle, E., 1994. Small intestinal digestion of starch in the horse. Revue Médecine Vétérinaire 145: 199-204.

Kienzle, E., Fehrle, S. and Opitz, B., 2002. Interactions between the Apparent Energy and Nutrient Digestibilities of a Concentrate Mixture and Roughages in Horses. The Journal of Nutrition.

Kienzle, E., Radicke, S., Landes, E., Kleffken, D., Illenseer, M. and Meyer, H., 1994. Activityof amylase in the gastrointestinal tract of the horse. Journal of Animal Physiol. Animal Nutrition 72: 234-241.

Kienzle, E. and Rainbird, A., 1991. The maintenance energy requirement of dogs - what is the correct figure for the calculation of the metabolic body weight in dogs? Journal of Nutrition 121: 39-40.

Kleiber, M., 1961. The Fire of Life. New York: John Wiley and Sons.
Kollarczik, B., Enders, C., Friedrich, M. and Gedek, B., 1992. Auswirkungen der Rations-zusammensetzung auf das Keimspektrum im Jejunum von Pferden (Effect of diet composition on microbial spectrum in the jejunum of horses). Pferdeheilkunde, Sonderausgabe, 49-54.
Lindemann, G., 1982. Untersuchungen über den Einfluß von Lactose- und Stärkezulagen auf die Verdaulichkeit von NH_3-aufgeschlossenem Stroh beim Pferd. Hannover, Tierärztliche Hochschule, Dissertation.
Löhlein, W., 1999, Untersuchungen zur Verdaulichkeit von Futtermitteln beim Asiatischen Elefanten (Elephas maximus). München, Tierärztliche Fakultät der Ludwig-Maximilians-Universität, Dissertation.
Lowman, R.S., Theodorou, M.K., Hyslopp, J.J., Dhanoa, M.S. and Cuddeford, D., 1999. Evaluation of an in vitro batch culture technique for estimating the in vivo digestibility and digestible energy content of equine feeds using equine feaces as the source of microbial inoculum. Animal Feed Science and Technology 80: 1, 11-27
McLean, B.M.L., Hyslopp, J.J., Longland, A.C., Cuddeford, D. and Hollands, T., 2000. Physical processing of barley and ist effects on intra-caecal fermentation parameters in ponies. Animal Feed Science and Technology 85: 1-2, 79-87
Meyer, H., Lindemann, G. and Schmidt, M., 1982. Einfluß unterschiedlicher Mischfuttergaben pro Mahlzeit auf praecaecale und postileale Verdauungsvorgänge beim Pferd. Fortschr. Tierphysiol. Tierernähr. Heft 13, 32-39.
Meyer, H., Radicke, S., Kienzle, E., Wilke, S. and Kleffken, D., 1993. Investigations on pre-ileal digestion of oats, corn, and barley starch in relation to grain processing. 13th Symposium Equine Nutrition Physiology, 21.-23.01.1993, Florida, Proceedings 43-48.
Meyer, H., Radicke, S., Kienzle, E., Wilke, S., Kleffken, D. and Illenseer, M., 1995. Investigation on praeileal digestion of starch from grain, potato and manioc in horses. J. Vet. Med, series A, 42(6): 371-381.
Pagan, D.J. and Hintz, H.F., 1986. Equine energetics. I. Relationship between body weight and energy requirements in horses. Journal of Animal Science, Bd. 63: 815-821.
Potter, G. D., Arnold F. F., Householder D. D., Hansen D. H., Brown K. M. (1992a): Digestion of starch in the small or large intestine of the equine. Pferdeheilkunde, Sonderheft 1.Europäische Konferenz über die Ernährung des Pferdes, Hannover, 107-111.
Potter G.D., Gibbs, P.G., Haley, R.G. and Klendshoj, C., 1992b. Digestion of protein in the small and large intestines of equines fed mixed diets. Pferdeheilkunde, Sonderausgabe, 140-143.
Schmidt, M., 1980. Untersuchungen über die Verträglichkeit und Verdaulichkeit eines pelletierten Mischfutters für Pferde in Kombination mit Heu und NH_3-aufgeschlossenem Stroh. Hannover, Tierärztliche Hochschule, Dissertation.
Schulze, K., 1987. Untersuchungen zur Verdaulichkeit und Energiebewertung von Mischfuttermitteln für Pferde. Hannover, Tierärztliche Hochschule, Dissertation.
Stillions, M.C. and Nelson. W.E., 1972. Digestible energy during maintenance of the light horse. Journal of Animal Science, Bd. 34: 981-982.
Wilke, S., 1992. Zur präilealen Verdaulichkeit von Hafer und Mais verschiedener Zubereitungen beim Pferd. Hannover, Tierärztliche Hochschule, Dissertation.
Zentek, J., Nyari, A. and Meyer, H., 1992. Untersuchungen zur postprandialen H_2- und CH_4-Exhalation beim Pferd (Investigations on postprandial H_2- and CH_4-exhaltion on the horse). Pferdeheilkunde, Sonderausgabe, 64-66.
Zeyner, A., 1995. Ermittlung des Gehaltes an verdaulicher Energie im Pferdefutter über die Verdaulichkeitsschätzung. Übers. Tierernährg. 23: 55-104.
Zeyner, A., 2002. Ernährungsphysiologische Wirkungen eines Austauschs von stärke-reichen Komponenten durch Sojaöl in der Reitpferdeernährung. Göttingen, Georg-August-Universität.
Zeyner, A. and Kienzle, E., 2001. ein neues Konzept zur energetischen Futterverwertung beim Pferd. Proc. Soc. Nutr. Physiol. 10: 106.
Zeyner, A. and Kienzle E., 2002. A Method to Estimate Digestible Energy in Horse Feed. The Journal of Nutrition.

Zeyner, A., Hoffmann, M. and Fuchs, R., 1992. Möglichkeiten zur Schätzung des Energiegehaltes in Rationen zur Sportpferdefütterung. Pferdeheilkunde Sonderausgabe, 175-178.

Zmija, G., 1991. Fütterungspraxis bei Galopp- und Trabrennpferden. Hannover, Tierärztliche Hochschule, Dissertation.

Evaluation and expression of energy allowances and energy value of feeds in the UFC system for the performance horse

W. Martin-Rosset and M. Vermorel

I.N.R.A. - Department of Animal Husbandry and Nutrition, Research Centre of Clermont-Ferrand/Theix, 63122 Saint-Genès Champanelle (France)

1. Introduction

The UFC system was developed by INRA in France (Vermorel et al., 1984; Vermorel and Martin-Rosset, 1997). This system provides sets of tables that give energy value of feeds and the nutrient requirements of horses (INRA, 1984-1990). Both are calculated as net energy and expressed in feed units, UFC (Unité Fourragère Cheval). The goals of this system in relation with the MADC system stated for protein (cf. Martin-Rosset and Tisserand's report in this issue) are to allow:

1) an accurate comparison of the nutritive value of feedstuffs;
2) the formulation of well balanced rations to achieve a production goal;
3) the prediction of the animal performance when amount and quality of rations are known.

The validity of the UFC system was tested through many feeding trials to state the new French feeding standards (Martin-Rosset et al., 1994).

This system is the official feeding standard in France (INRA, 1990) and it is used in an increasing number of European Countries with or without local adaptation (Miraglia and Olivieri, 1990; Staun, 1990; Smolders, 1990; Austbø, 1996 and see Ellis' report in this issue).

This paper gives the main figures used for stating the UFC system: 1) energy metabolism and requirements of the performance horse (young and adult), 2) evaluation of the energy value of feedstuffs used to meet the requirements, 3) evaluation and expression of energy recommended allowances.

2. Evaluation, expression, and prediction of the energy value of feeds

2.1 Origin of the French net energy system

From the results of feeding trials on draught horses, German workers proposed a feed evaluation system for horses based on the net energy (NE) value of feeds for work more than a century ago (Wolff and Kreuzhage, 1895). NE for work was the energy content of feeds which contributed to meeting energy expenditure of working horses. However, because of lack of information on feed digestion and energy utilization in horses, this system dropped to the benefit of existing systems based on digestible energy (DE) and net energy for fattening in ruminants.

Thanks to increased knowledge on feed digestibility and digestion in horses, and energy utilization for various functions in ruminants and pigs, and for fattening (Fingerling quoted by Nehring and Francke, 1954; in Francke, 1954; Hoffmann et al., 1967; Willard et al., 1979; Kane et al., 1979) or maintenance (Hintz, 1968) in horses, a new NE system was concieved and introduced in France (Vermorel et al., 1984). It was further improved by taking into account the results obtained in horses and ponies at INRA (Vermorel and Martin-Rosset, 1997). Its validity was tested in light horses fed twelve diferent diets, using energy balances determined by indirect calorimetry

(Vermorel et al., 1997), and the results of many feeding trials performed at INRA on mares, growing horses and working horses (Martin-Rosset et al., 1994). The energy value of feeds and the energy allowances for horses are expressed in the same unit, the ''horse feed unit'' (UFC).

2.2 Structure of the French NE system

The NE value of feeds is calculated through a step-wise procedure from 1) the gross energy (GE) content, 2) the energy digestibility (ED) as measured in horses, 3) the ratio between ME and DE as determined in horses, 4) the assumed proportions of absorbed energy supplied by the various nutrients, 5) the efficiencies of ME utilization for maintenance (km) of the main nutrients:
NE = ME x km or NE = GE x ED x ME/DE x km

In addition, the NE content of feeds is related to that of a reference feed (barley), and expressed in ''horse feed unit'' (Unité Fourragère Cheval, UFC)
UFC value of a feed = NE content of feed / NE content of barley

2.3 Metabolisable energy of feeds

Gross energy can be determined using a bomb calorimeter or predicted from the feed chemical composition, with a residual standard deviation (RSD) of 0.5% (Vermorel and Martin-Rosset, 1997).

Organic matter digestibility (OMD) of 33 forages was determined in horses and in sheep. Relationships were computed between OMD in horses and OMD in sheep with RSDs of 2.3 to 2.6 percent units. Most OMD of concentrate feeds were obtained in horses. The missing OMDs were drawn from either pig tables (for feeds with less than 15% CF) or extrapolated from pig and ruminant tables (Martin-Rosset et al., 1984).

Energy digestibility (ED) of 75 feeds was measured in horses in France and in the Netherlands. A relationship was calculated to predict ED from OMD, with a RSD of 1.1 percent unit (Martin-Rosset et al., 1994).

Metabolisable energy: Methane and urinary energy were determined in light horses fed 12 different diets at one or two feeding levels. However, the number of data was insufficient to predict methane and urinary energy losses of the various feeds. Therefore, a relationship was established from the 79 available data to predict ME from DE, with a RSD of 1.37 percent unit (Vermorel and Martin-Rosset, 1997).

2.4 Prediction of nutrient supply

The NE value of a feed depends on the amounts of the various nutrients absorbed from the digestive tract and the individual efficiency of energy utilisation for ATP production. For feeds of similar DE the nutrient supply may vary depending on chemical composition, and site and type of digestion (enzymatic digestion in the small intestine with production of glucose, aminoacids and long chain fatty acids, or fermentation in the large intestine with production of volatile fatty acids, VFA, methane and fermentation heat).

The amounts of nutrients supplied by the various feeds were estimated from the results obtained in digestion studies with fistulated horses or in slaugther experiments. Due to lack of information for some feeds, several hypotheses were made, based on knowledge of digestion in pigs and ruminants. Energy losses as methane and fermentation heat were taken into account. The amounts of energy supplied by the various nutrients were estimated from their individual gross energy content. Such estimates were made for 95 feeds (various forages, beets and beet pulp, cereals, cereal by-products and oil meals). It is noticeable that glucose (+ lactate) supplies 64% of absorbed energy from maize grain and 10% from poor quality hay, whereas VFA supply only 20% of absorbed energy from maize but 75-80% from poor quality hay (Vermorel and Martin-Rosset, 1997).

2.5 Efficiency of ME utilisation for maintenance and work

In resting and exercising horses energy requirements result mainly from free-energy (e.g. ATP) utilization for maintenance (metabolic and physiological processes such as ions and molecules transport accross membranes to maintain concentration gradients, substrate cycles, protein and phospholipids turnover..., secretion, excretion, gut motility, blood circulation...and muscle tonus), on one hand, and for physical activity (muscle contraction, increases in calcium transport, heart and other muscle activity), on the other hand. Therefore, the NE value of feeds has been estimated from their ATP production potential (Vermorel and Martin-Rosset, 1997). The latter cannot be directly determined because most free-energy is lost as heat during ATP utilization. However, it can be estimated by a biochemical approach (Armstrong, 1969, among others). It is noticeable that this concept has recently been proposed to evaluate the NE value of feeds for humans (Livesey, 2001).

In fasting animals free-energy is drawn from the oxidative catabolism of body reserves, mainly lipids. Therefore, the NE value of a feed for maintenance is defined as its energy content which contributes to spare body reserves in a fasting animal. The biochemical efficiency of nutrients energy utilization for ATP production is 38% for lipids, 40% for glucose, 34% for the usual VFA mixture and 31% for protein. Consequently, the NE value of nutrients compared to that of body lipids is 100% for glucose, 95% for lipids, 84% for VFA, and 78% for protein. These estimates were confirmed by the results obtained in fasting rats, dogs, ruminants and ponies fed pure nutrients.

In working animals the free-energy used for physical activity is also mainly drawn from body reserves (first muscle glycogen and lipid droplets, then liver glycogen and adipose tissue lipids), especially in the performance horse, and to a lesser extent from nutrients.**The efficiencies of ATP production from various energy substrates are the same for work and for maintenance**. However, the efficiency of ATP utilisation to perform mechanical work (external work) is low, 55% maximum, and decreases with increasing muscle contraction speed (see infra). This explains why the net efficiency of ME utilisation for mechanical (external) work is low and averages 25% in draught horses (Brody, 1945) and decreases when the speed increases (see infra).

These differences in efficiency of ME (or nutrient energy) utilization for maintenance and for work are confusing for people who are not familiar with energy metabolism. However, it must be reminded that the efficiency of ME (or nutrient energy) utilization for ATP production is the same for maintenance and for work. ***This means that feeds (or nutrients) have the same relative energy value for maintenance and for work,*** even if large differences are known to exist between the absolute values. Consequently, the **UFC values of feeds are the same for maintenance and work**. This underlines the interest of expressing the NE value of feeds in feed units (UFC), that is the NE value of a feed relative to that of barley, rather than their NE value in kJ.
Maintenance was chosen as the reference situation to estimate the NE value of feeds because maintenance accounts for 70-80% of total energy expenditure in working horses, 90-60% in growing horses (Martin-Rosset et al., 1994), and 50-90% in lactating and pregnant mares (Martin-

Rosset and Doreau, 1984; Doreau et al., 1988). The overestimation of efficiency of ME utilization for work, growth or lactation was compensated for by increases in energy requirements.

2.5.1 Energy cost of eating

Several studies carried out in horses and ponies showed that the energy cost of eating per kg DM of feed was 2 to 3 times higher in horses than in ruminants (Vermorel and Mormède, 1991; Vernet et al., 1995; Vermorel et al., 1996) because horses spent twice as much time chewing forages as ruminants (Doreau, 1978). The measured efficiency of ME utilisation of 6 hays was 4% units lower than expected from the energy utilisation of nutrients (Vernet et al., 1995). Therefore, a correction factor was computed which depended on energy didestibility or crude fibre content of forages.

2.5.2 Calculation of ME efficiency (km)

Km (%) is calculated from the assumed quantities of nutrients supplied during digestion, their gross energy content (E), the individual efficiencies of energy utilisation for maintenance, and the correction factor for the energy cost of eating forages, using the following relationships:

For forages:

$$km = 0.85\ EGl + 0.80\ ELCFA + 0.70\ EAA + (0.63 \text{ to } 0.68)\ EAGV - 0.14\ (76.4 - ED) \text{ or}$$

$$km = 0.85\ EGl + 0.80\ ELCFA + 0.70\ EAA + (0.63 \text{ to } 0.68)\ EAGV - 0.20\ CF + 2.50$$

For concentrate feeds:

$$km = 0.85\ EGl + 0.80\ ELCFA + 0.70\ EAA + (0.63 \text{ to } 0.68)\ EAGV$$

where E is the percentage of absorbed energy supplied by glucose and lactate (Gl), long chain fatty acids (LCFA), aminoacids (AA) and volatile fatty acids (VFA); ED is energy digestibility (%) and CF the crude fibre content (%).

km ranged from 80% for maize to 66-62% for hays and 45-43% for straw.

2.6 NE value of feeds

The NE content (MJ/ kg) of a feed is calculated from its ME content and the efficiency of ME utilization for maintenance: NE = ME x km.

The NE content of standard barley, the reference feed, is 9.42 MJ / kg

One ''horse feed unit'' (1 UFC) corresponds to 9.42 MJ NE for maintenance

The NE value of common feeds ranges from 1.15 UFC (maize) to 0.54-0.35 (hays)

2.6.1 Prediction of the UFC value of simple feeds

The UFC value of 95 feeds was calculated as described previously. Relationship were computed between the UFC values and the chemical composition, with or without DOM or DE as independent variables. Using cytoplasmic carbohydrates as independent variate reduced RSD to 0.032 UFC/kg DM. Adding DOM or DE as independent variate reduced RSD to 0.012 and 0.017 UFC/kg DM for forages and concentrates, respectively (Vermorel and Martin-Rosset, 1997).

2.6.2 Prediction of the UFC value of compound feeds

The UFC value of 15 compound feeds of known composition (open formula) was calculated as described before. Relationships were computed between their UFC value and their chemical composition as determined by routine analysis. The lowest RSD (0.031 UFC/kg OM) was obtained with starch and the Van Soest analysis components as independant variables.

2.7 Tests of the validity of the UFC system

The validity of several assumptions and hypotheses used in the UFC system have been tested during the last decade.

Digestibility studies carried out with light horses showed that OMD and ED were not significantly altered by feeding level and that there were no significant forage-concentrate interaction whatever the feeding level (Martin-Rosset and Dulphy, 1987; Martin-Rosset et al., 1990).

The energy utilization of 12 diets expected to give large variations in the proportions of digestion end-products was determined in light horses. There was a good agreement between the experimental and the predicted values of km since the differences averaged only 0.6 +/ - 1.2% (Vermorel et al., 1997).

The UFC value of 21 commercial compound feeds of known composition representative of compound feeds used in Europe was estimated using the previous prediction equations. The differences between the predicted UFC values and those calculated by addition averaged 0.004 + /- 0.016 UFC/kg OM, which shows that the UFC value of compound feeds can be predicted accurately from their chemical composition determined by routine analysis (Martin-Rosset et al., 1996a).

2.8. Routine prediction of the UFC value of feedstuffs in the UFC system

The UFC value of feedstuffs can be routinely predicted:

- using a set of tables performed for horses (INRA 1990)
  The UFC values of 150 feedstuffs (forages + concentrates: e.g. ingredients) are proposed. The UFC values can be read directly for forages when species, stage and conditions at harvest are known. Similarly the UFC value of ingredients can be read directly if the ingredients have not been subjected to sophisticated processes.
- from the results of laboratory analysis using sets of equations (table 1) and a panel of lab methods (Martin-Rosset 1996 a). The UFC value of forages can be predicted from analytical criteria measured with chemical, enzymatic and physical methods performed by INRA (Andrieu and Martin-Rosset, 1995; Martin-Rosset 1996 b and 1996 c; Andrieu et al., 1996; Martin-Rosset, 2001).

2.9 Interest of the UFC system

The UFC system is an empirical model which does not pretend to predict the ''true'' energy values of feeds, but to approach them closer than a DE system. It takes into account differences in methane and energy losses and differences in ME utilization for maintenance between feeds. Comparing cereals and hays, this results in further differences of 8% between DE and ME, and 18 to 28% between ME and NE. Thus, the UFC value of 1 kg DM of a medium quality hay is 32% that of 1kg DM of maize, whereas the DE value is 49%. The UFC system gives a better estimate of the energy value of forages than a DE system.

The main limit of accuracy of the UFC system is the estimate of the percentages of absorbed energy supplied by the main nutrients. However, errors in these estimates have relatively small effects on km (Vermorel and Martin-Rosset, 1997). Finally, contrary to some unfounded assertions, using km to estimate the UFC value of feeds for maintenance and work does not introduce any bias since nutrients energy or ME are used with the same efficiency to produced ATP used either for maintenance processes or for physical activity.

Table 1. Prediction equations of the UFC value of feeds for horses from chemical composition and digestible organic matter or digestible energy content (from Martin-Rosset et al., 1994 and 1996a, Vermorel and Martin-Rosset 1997).

	RSD	R^2
2.a - Forages (n = 47)		
N° 2.1 UFC = 0.825 -1.090 CF + 0.555 CP	0.043	0.832
N°2.2 UFC=0.568-0.650CF +0.687CP+1.804CC	0.031	0.922
N° 2.3 UFC = - 0.124 + 0.254 CC + 1.330 DOM	0.012	0.988
N°2.4 UFC=-0.056 +0.562 CC +0.0619 DE	0.007	0.996
2.b - Concentrates; Raw materials (n = 51)		
N ° 2.5 UFC = 0.815 - 0.947 CF + 0.0345 CP + 0.582 CC	0.060	0.931
N° 2.6 UFC = 0.131- 0.628 CF - 0.282 CP + 1.340 DOM	0.041	0.967
N° 2.7 UFC = - 0.730 - 0.722 CP + 0.572 OM + 0.0941 DE	0.033	0.979
N°2.8 UFC=-0.134+0.274CF-0.362CP+0.316CC+0.0755DE	0.017	0.995
2.c - Compound feeds		
N° 2.9 UFCo =1.326 -1.937 CFo - 0.135 Cpo	0.060	0.956
N° 2.10 UFCo =1.333 -1.684 ADFo - 0.096 Cpo	0.060	0.958
N° 2.11 UFCo =1.173 -1.605 CFo + 0.051 CPo + 0.215 STAo	0.043	0.976
N° 2.12 UFCo =1.181 -1.397 ADFo + 0.082 CPo + 0.214 STAo	0.040	0.978
N° 2.13 UFCo =1.219 - 0.852 ADFo - 0.287 NDFo - 0.857 Llo + 0.034 CPo+ 0.207 STAo	0.031	0.988

Abbreviations and units
UFC: horse feed unit (per kg DM); UFCo = horse feed unit (per kg OM)
DM: dry matter OM: organic matter; CF: crude fibre; CP: crude protein;
CC: cytoplasmic carbohydrates (water soluble carbohydrates + starch);
ADF: acid detergent fibre; NDF: neutral detergent fibre
} (kg per kg dry matter)
CFo, CPo, etc... expressed in kg per kg organic matter.
DOM: digestible organic matter (kg/kg DM);
DE: digestible energy (MJlkg DM)

3. Evaluation and expression of energy requirements and recommanded allowances of the performance horse

3.1 Definitions and methods for determination

In France, nutrient requirements and allowances are clearly distinguished. The requirements stand for physiological expenditure of horses for maintenance, growth and exercise. The requirements are met by the nutrients of the ration, and by body reserves when the amount of nutrients supplied is inadequate. The nutrient allowances are the amounts of nutrients provided by the ration. A recommended allowance is the amount of nutrients which should be supplied to horses to achieve a desirable level of performance allowed by their potential. The animals are assumed to be in good health, well managed and housed during the winter period. These should be considered as optimum allowances, which meet at least the requirements. Exceptions are:

- growing horses bred for school-riding or hacking where limited growth is assumed during the winter period, but a compensatory growth period is expected during the subsequent summer period to achieve an optimum body weight at late bracking (figure 1)

- exercising horses where a moderate and controlled use of body reserves is assumed at short term (a few days) during the training period to avoid physiopathologic disorders related to large variation in workload and subsequent daily nutrient intake.

Energy allowances have been estimated either by a factorial method from metabolic data and/or by feeding experiments depending on the physiological function. With the factorial method, the amount of energy deposited or exported was divided by the metabolic efficiencies of energy, which are specific to the physiological function. With the feeding method, the allowances have been determined by long-term feeding trials conducted with a great number of horses.

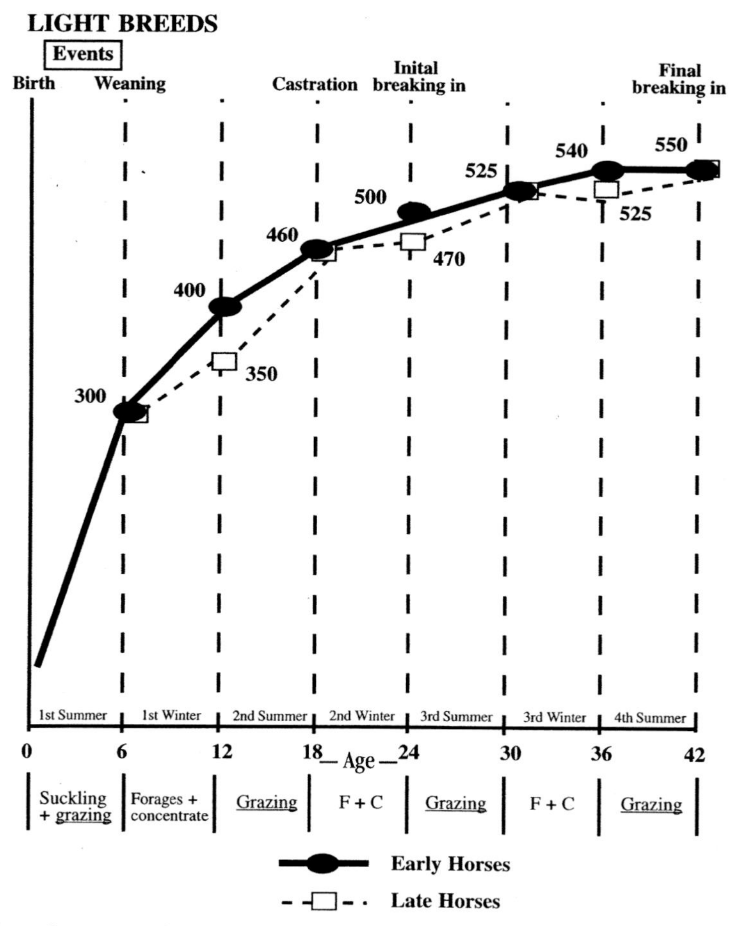

Figure 1. Growth curve and management of young sport horses (selle français or anglo-arabe) established from INRA long term feeding experiments (from INRA 1990).

3.2 Energy expenditure, efficiency of substrates energy utilisation and energy requirements for maintenance and work

3.2.1 Variations of energy expenditure

Mean daily energy expenditure of horses varies with physical and physiological characteristics and physical activity of the animals. It can be roughly considered as the sum of the maintenance energy expenditure and the increase in energy expenditure associated with exercise although the two components are not independent.

3.2.2 Maintenance

Maintenance is the main component of daily energy expenditure and accounts for 50 to 80% of that of a working horse.

Maintenance energy expenditure is proportionnal to metabolic body weight (MBW) as it was stated from feeding trials and indirect calorimetry studies (cf. Review of Martin-Rosset et al., 1994). The maintenance energy expenditure per kg MBW also varies with other factors linked to the horse and its environnement.

Individual variations (per kg MBW) measured in horses at rest are a good indicator of mettle; the range of variation is 10 to 20% on average (Hoffmann et al., 1967; Wooden et al., 1970; Martin-Rosset and Vermorel, 1991).Variations are probably related to differences in tissue metabolic rate, muscle tone and spontaneous physical activity.

The effect of breed is probalby linked to some extend to the effect of mettle. Light breed horses display energy expenditure 20% higher on average than heavy breeds and poneys (Nadal'jak, 1961; Vermorel et al., 1997). To our knowledge, the variability between light breeds has not been studied.

The effect of sex must be allowed for, since the maintenance requirements have been found to be 10-15% greater in males than in gelding and females (Anderson et al., 1983; Axelsson, 1949; Breuer, 1968; Brody, 1945; Kossila et al., 1972; Stillions and Nelson, 1972).

Increases in feeding level can elevate maintenance energy expenditure as well (Kellner, 1909; Martin-Rosset and Vermorel, 1991) because of the high metabolic rate of gut tissues and liver.

Effect of climatic conditions:the maintenance energy expenditure is on average 10% higher in summer than in winter in the temperate zones (Martin-Rosset and Vermorel, 1991). Under the low critical temperature: -15 °C (Cymbaluck and Christison 1990), energy expenditure would be increased by 2.5% $°C^{-1}$ (Mc Bride et al., 1985).

Comparing horse at rest and in *training* Kellner, 1909 demonstrated using feeding trials, that maintenance energy expenditure was higher in exercising horses than in resting horses. This effect could result from an extended stimulation of the sympathetic nervous system as shown in humans.

Finally *transportation* of horses by road increases energy expenditure of resting horses: 3.0 J vs 1.3 J kg^{-1} s^{-1} (Doherty et al., 1997).

3.2.3 Work

When a horse moves, its energy expenditure exceeds its maintenance requirement. This additionnal expenditure results first from the work done by skeletal muscles, and secondly from the increased work done by the respiratory, cardiovascular system and other organs, and the increased tone of all the other skeletal muscles.

Oxygen consumption is the best criterium of energy expenditure. It was measured in laboratory conditions in horses exercising on a treadmill (Brody et al., 1945; Hoffman et al., 1967) and later in more natural conditions, with increasingly elaborated equipment, in horses pulling a load (Brody, 1945), harnessed to a sulky (Karlsen and Nadal'jak, 1964) and finally saddled (Hornicke et al., 1974, 1983; Meixner et al., 1981; Pagan and Hintz, 1986).

The oxygen consumption (about 3 ml/min/kg live weight at rest) increases linearly with speed up to gallop (550 m/min) for saddlle horse with riders (figure 2). At the highest speeds studied (600 to 700 m/ min), the oxygen consumption averages 100 ml/min/kg. In well trained horses, the maximum oxygen consumption may reach 125 to 140 ml/min/kg liveweight. At this peak level, the anaerobic metabolism predominates and energy expenditure is higher than expected from oxygen consumption. Indeed, the latter remains high after the effort ceases, and return gradually to the rest level. This additionnal oxygen consumption (oxygen debt) must be added to the amount of oxygen consumed during exercice. Consequently, at the higest speeds, energy expenditure increases exponentially with speed (figure 3). However, importantly when the oxygen consumed is expressed relative to the distance travelled and not the time elapsed, it is not dependent on velocity (Hornicke et al., 1983): 0.21 ml/kg/m at a walking pace and 0.19 at a trot.
The energy expenditure was calculated from the measurement of oxygen consumption multiplied by the thermal equivalent of 0_2 corresponding to the RQ (respiratory quotient) calculated at each measurement point (Brody, 1945).

At a walking pace, the energy cost (e.g. total expenditure - expenditure at rest) ranges from 1.4 to 1.6 J/kg BW/m for horizontal locomotion at 80 -à 100 m/min (Zuntz and Hageman, 1898). As a

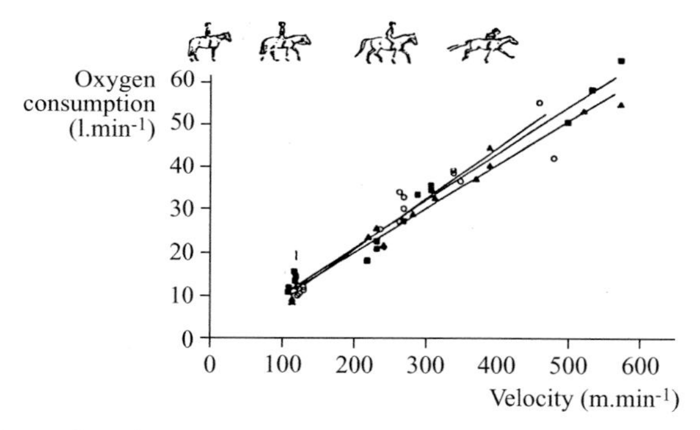

Figure 2. Relationships between oxygen consumption (VO_2) and velocity (V) in sports horses (from Meixner, Hörnicke, Ehrlein, 1981).

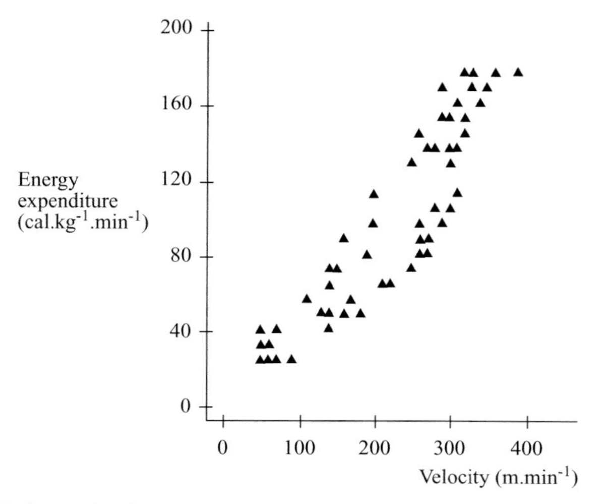

Figure 3. Relationship between energy expended (D) and velocity (V) (from Pagan and Hintz, 1986b).

result the daily energy expenditure was increased by 18 to 36 p 100 (e.g. 7%/h) by 12 and 24 km walks, respectively (Hoffmann et al., 1967). The energy expenditure of a walking horse is 8 times higher at a velocity of 180 m/min than at rest (figure 3). In addition, the energy cost of walking is multiplied by 2.5 when slope rises to 10% (Zuntz and Hageman, 1898; Anderson et al., 1983). The energy cost of the vertical elevation when the horse is jumping is 15 fold higher (29 kJ/kg BW/m) than that at horizontal locomotion.

3.2.4 Trot and gallop

The energy cost of horizontal locomotion would increase fro 1.2 to 2.3 J/kg/m (e.g. + 53%) when the horse begins trotting at the same velocity (100 m/mn) (Zuntz and Hagemann, 1898). The energy expenditure of horses increases exponentially with speed at fast trot and gallop, from 10 times resting energy expenditure at a slow trot (200/m/min) to 40 folds at a fast gallop (600 m/min) and about 60 folds at top velocity (table 2) because the efficiency of energy utilisation falls (figures 3, 4) since the anaerobic glycolysis predominates.

3.2.5 Energy efficiency

Although the energy efficiency has been studied mainly in draught work (Brody, 1945), the results clearly illustrate how energy utilization depends on the intensity of effort.

Energy efficiency is defined as the ratio between the work done (in Joules) and the corresponding energy expenditure (in Joules). The work done is the external work performed (kgm) multiplied by the thermal equivalent (1 kgm = 9.81 J). Energy expenditure is calculated from oxygen consumption (including oxygen debt) and the thermal equivalent of O_2 for the corresponding RQ.

Table 2. Variations of the energy expenditure with the velocity in the horse[1]: unit energy cost (from INRA 1984).

Situation	Velocity (m/mn)	Energy expenditure	
		(Kcal/mn)	Times of maintenance (maintenance = 1)
Waiting without rider	0	11.5	1.1
Waiting with rider	0	12	1.2
Walk	110	50	2.5
Slow trot	200	110	10
Normal trot	300	160	15
Fast trot[2]	500	350	35
Normal galop	350	210	20
Fast galop[2]	600	420	40
Maximum velocity[2]		600	60

[1] The energy expenditures were calculated from the oxygen consumption (and oxygen debt) measured by Meixner, Hornicke and Ehrlein (1981) in horses of 560 kg body weight carrying a load of 100 kg (rider + hack + apparatus). For walk, energy expenditure was calculated from datas of Brody, 1945, Hoffmann et al., 1967, Nadal'Jak, 1961, Zuntz and Hagemann, 1898

[2] Value calculated from the maximum oxygen consumption of horses estimate by Vermorel Jarrige and Martin-Rosset 1984 and the oxygen debt

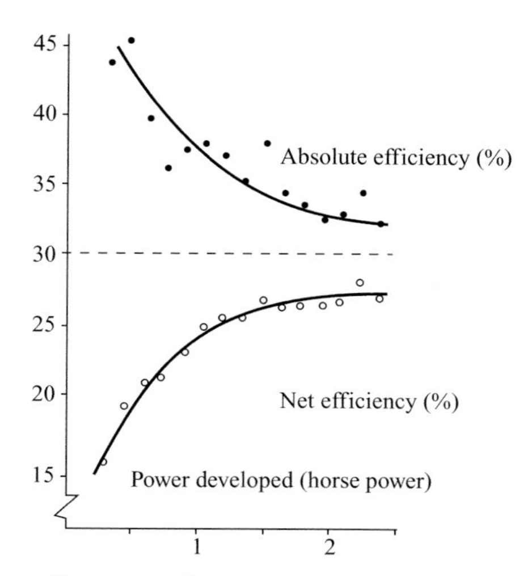

Figure 4. Absolute energy efficiency and net energy in horses versus horse power (from Brody, 1945).

Energy efficiency can be expressed as *net efficiency* or *absolute efficiency*.

Net efficiency is the ratio between work performed (kJ) and energy expended for locomotion and work above that at rest:

- *Net effeciency* = Work performed / (Total energy expended during work - resting energy expenditure)

Absolute efficiency is the ratio between work performed (kJ) and energy expended above that of locomotion without load, e.g. energy expended for work only:

- *Absolute efficiency* = Work performed / (Total energy expended during work - Energy expended during locomotion without load)

The net efficiency of energy utilization for work decreases with increasing velocity and tends asymptotically to 28% (figure 4). Similarly the *absolute efficiency* decreases from 45 to 30%. This results from 1) the low efficiency of anaerobic glycolysis, 2) the drop of mechanical effiency of ATP utilization for muscle contraction from 50 to 17% (Kushmerick and Davies, 1969), and 3) the utilization of energy for other purposes such as respiration, blood circulation and the increase in tone of other skeletal muscles. In fact, only 35% of energy expended above that at rest is used for the so- called external work (Brody, 1945).

The efficiency of energy utilisation for physical activity varies also with *other factors*. The net efficiency for horizontal locomotion with or without load falls when the horse trots rather than walking (table 3). In addition, the net efficiency decreases by 25 or 33% when the slope rises from 0 to 8% in horses pulling a load at walk or at a trot, respectively. In other respects, the net efficiency tends to be lower in trotters than in draught horses. Lastly, there are wide individual variations among horses probably depending on physical capacities, training status, and climatic conditions.

Table 3. Average net efficiencies in horses (from Grandeau and Alekan, 1904 (a), Brody 1945 (b), Nadal'jack 1961 (c).

Efficiency (%)	Gait	
	Walk	Trot
Harnessed horses (a)	20-25	13-16
Trotters (c)	14-19	9
Heavy horses (b, c)	18-25	12

3.3 Energy requirements of young horses

Body composition of young horses varies with age since the proportions of the different tissues changes. Drawn from data obtained in heavy breeds, the proportion of muscle decrases from 51 to 40% during the breeding period (without training), whereas the proportion of adipose tissues rises from 8 to 10%, and the proportion of bone tissues decreases from 11 to 10% (Martin-Rosset et al., 1983b). As a result, the chemical composition of the empty body weight gain changes between weaning to 2 years of age (figure 5): The lipid content increases sharply (from 0 to 40%). In addition, it varies markedly according to the average daily gain (from - 5 to + 16%; table 4).
In light breeds, the energy content of body weight gain increases sharply from 4.8 MJ to 8.9 MJ /kg between 320 (yearling) and 470 kg (2 year old) of body weight for 0.5 Kg daily gain. In addition, when daily gain varies from 0.5 to 1.0 Kg, energy content of body weigth gain increase from 4.8 to 12.8MJ at 320 kg body weight (yearling).

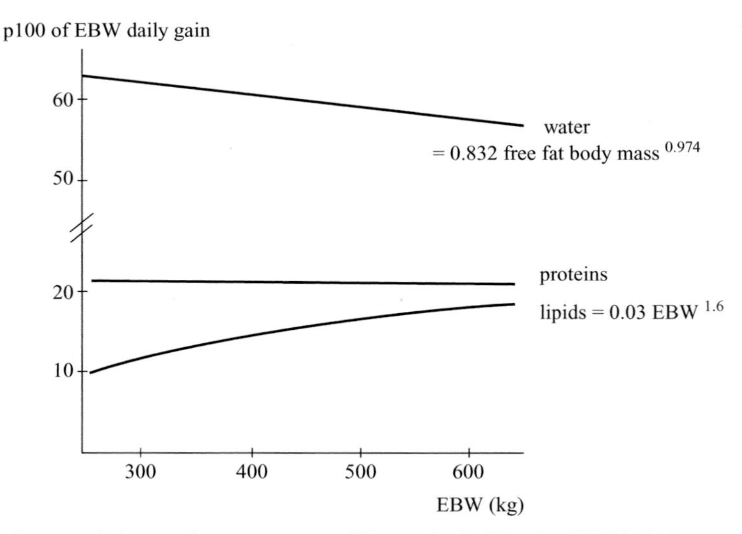

Figure 5. Evolution of chemical composition of Empty body Weight (EBW) daily gain between 6 to 30 months (drawn from Agabriel et al., 1984).

Table 4. Chemical composition of daily gain in yearling and long yearling of breed in different situations (drawn from Agabriel et al., 1984).

Type of animal	Daily gain of BW[1] g/d	Daily gain of EBW[1] g/d	Chemical composition of EBW[1] daily gain		Chemical composition of BW[1] daily gain		
			Lipids p.100	Protein p.100	Lipids p.100	Protein p.100	Energy Cal.
Yearling (6-12 months)							
• 1st trial [2]	1100	890	13	20.9	10.6	16.9	1890
• 2nd trial [3]	500	400	- 5.5	25.2	- 4.4	20.2	825 [4]
	1000	800	11.3	21.1	9.0	16.9	1720
	1390	1100	15.9	19.7	12.6	15.6	2060
Long Yearling (12-18 months)							
Growth during the prior winter							
• slow		950	8-11	21-22			
• moderate		840	2-6	23-24			

[1] BW = Body Weight EBW = Empty Body Weight
[2] Average values observed in yearlings fed with the same diet: anatomical composition was measured by dissection of half carcass
[3] Referenced values obtained when comparing yearlings affected by different feeding levels: anatomical composition was predicted from anatomical dissection of the 14th rib according to Martin-Rosset et al., 1985.
[4] Lipids content was considered to be 0

3.4 Energy recommended allowances

In horses, as in other farm animals, a distinction between maintenance and production requirements has been made, although the overall metabolism is influenced by variations in animal energy expenditures.

3.4.1 INRA recommended allowances

- *Maintenance*

These have been assessed from former feeding standards and the results of recent feeding trials. They average 588 kJ DE/kg MBW or 504 kJ ME/kg MBW, thus 353 kJ NE/kg MBW or 0.038 UFC/kg MBW (Vermorel et al., 1984). These requirements were checked using the results of feeding and calorimetry trials in horses of light breeds (Martin-Rosset and Vermorel, 1991). The daily NE requirements average 36.96 MJ and 48.05 MJ for geldings weighing 500 and 700 kg, respectively. In addition, the maintenance requirements are increased by 5 to 10% for sports horses and bloodstocks, respectively, and by 15 or 20% for stallions of sports breeds and bloodstock, respectively. For working horses allowances are increased by 5 to 15% to take into account the rise of the overall energy metabolism (Kellner, 1909) and the importance of spontaneous activities related to temper in exercising horses.

- *Work*

Two methods can be used to evaluate energy requirements or allowances for work: the **factorial** (analytical) **method** and the **global method** (feeding experiments). The factorial method requires the accurate measurement of duration, intensity and energy cost of each type of physical activity, and the estimate of the ancillary effects (anticipation and remanence).The global method consists in measuring the quantity of energy required by adult horses to maintain constant body weight and condition in various situations. This is the most satisfactory method both in practice and from a physiological standpoint, because it takes into account all variables. However, it requires the determination of the nutritive value of feeds, feed intake, and variations in horse body reserves, which is seldom done. Furthermore, it is applicable only in well defined situations.

In the INRA system the factorial method has been used to estimate the energy cost of a standard hour of very light, light, moderate or intense work from the duration and nature of the physical activities (walk, ordinary trot, ordinary gallop, jumps) and their unitary unit costs (table 2). The energy expenditure was loaded to take into account the ancillary effects of anticipation and remanence. This loading (10 to 20%), can only be very approximate in the current state of knowledge.

The reliability of these estimates has been tested through feeding trials carried out over 6- month-periods at the National Riding School of Saumur, France (n = 80 horses), and at the Animal Technology Teaching Centre of Rambouillet, France (n = 24 horses of the equine section). The energy requirements were estimated as described above, and taking into account the body weight of horses and the work performed (duration, velocity). Feed intake was determined individually, and the net energy value of the rations had been determined (digestibility and indirect calorimetry; Vermorel et al., 1997). Variations of body weight and body composition were also taken into account (INRA, 1990; Martin-Rosset et al., 1991; INRA - HN - IE, 1998 and Martin-Rosset et al., in preparation). The feed allowances were of the same order of magnitude as the requirements calculated by the analytical method, allowing for the ancillary effects. These results show that the method used is good, and the energy allowances recommended in 1984 and updated in 1990 are satisfactory (figure 6).

The energy requirements for work are additional to the maintenance requirements of horses at rest. Requirements and allowances of energy in the horse are expressed in UFC (INRA, 1984; Martin-Rosset et al., 1994). For practical reasons, and in particular to forestall rationing errors, recommended energy allowances tables (maintenance plus work) have been drawn up for the situations most often encountered by sports and leisure horses of different sizes (table 5). In these tables, the energy figures are given alongside the recommended allowances for protein and minerals. These tables are used directly to calculate rations.

- *Growth*

These requirements have been evaluated from feeding trials (Agabriel et al., 1984; Bigot et al., 1987; Micol and Martin-Rosset, 1995) in which NE (UFC) intake, body weight and weight gain of young horses were precisely measured, for three reasons:

1) The energy requirement for maintenance (per kg MBW) varies with breed and growth rate. The variations in maintenance requirements due to breed are known only in adults. The amount of energy retained per kg body weight gain computed from the chemical composition of tissues has been determined only in heavy breeds (Martin-Rosset et al., 1983b).
2) The efficiency of metabolizable energy utilization for growth is not know yet.

Energy allowances were computed according to body weight (BW) and weight gain (G) of young horses using a relationship established from the results of feeding trials carried out at INRA, and according to the following model set up for growing bulls (Geay et al., 1978; Robelin, 1979):
$UFC/kg\ MBW/day = a + bG^{1.4}$
a = coefficient of maintenance requirement; G = average daily gain (kg/day)

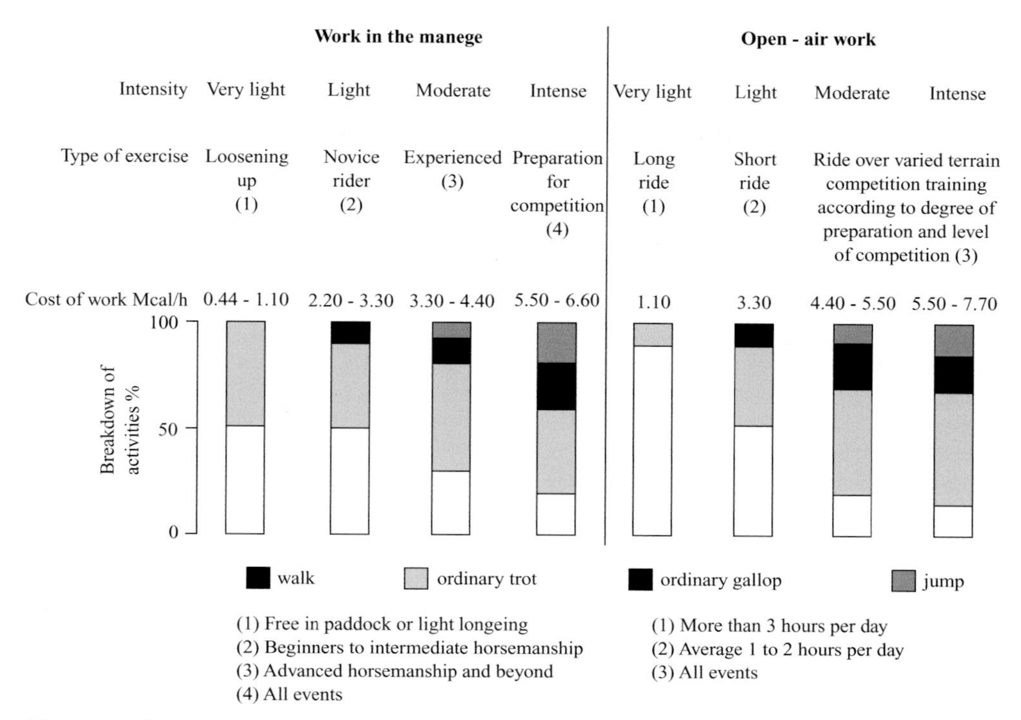

Figure 6. Approximate evaluation of energy cost per hour of work done by a sports horse according the nature and duration of the work, additionnal to daily maintenance requirements (from INRA, 1984 and 1990; Martin-Rosset et al., 1994).

The validity of the model and namely of the exponent “1.4” was checked in horses from the results of slaughter experiments in young heavy horses and extended to light breeds (Agabriel et al., 1984).

The relationships obtained for growing horses of light breeds are given in table 6. For 1 kg daily gain, the total daily net energy requirement amounts to 45.3 MJ at 250 kg BW and 59.1 MJ at 350 kg BW, because of increases in both maintenance requirement (+10.16 MJ) and in energy deposited (+ 3.70 MJ/kg). Since the energy content of body gain varies with growth rate, **two levels of allowances** were proposed according to the production goal (horses produced for school riding and hacking or bloodstock produced for competition) and the growth potential of the young horses.

3.4.2 Comparison of energy requirements expressed in UFC (INRA, 1984 - 1990) and in DE (NRC, 1989)

Energy requirements for maintenance, growth, and work have been expressed in% of maintenance requirements in both systems (table 7). The relative requirements are similar in yearlings, lower in 2 year- old and in working horses in the NRC than in the INRA systems. In other respects, direct comparison have been made of energy requirements expressed in DE in both systems. In the NRC system maintenance requirements of mature horses is 10% higher than in the INRA system. Total requirements of yearlings are similar (100 and 108%) but lower in the NRC system than in the INRA system for 2 year-old horses (71% for rapid growth) and for working horses (90 and 95% for moderate and intense exercise).

Table 5. Recommended daily energy (UFC or Mcal NE) and nitrogen (MADC) allowances for exercising sport and leisure horses of light breed (500 kg mature liveweight) (INRA, 1990).

Use	Daily allowances [1]							Daily Feed * (kg DM **)
	UFC	NE (Mcal)	MADC (g)	Ca (g)	P (g)	Mg (g)	Na (g)	
Maintenance:								
Horse at rest	4.2	9.73	295	25	15	7	12	7.0-8.5
Work								
Very light [2,4]	5.4	11.88	370	28	16	8	22	8.5-9.5
Light [2,4]	6.9	15.18	470	30	18	9	37	9.5-11.5
Moderate [2,4]	7.9	17.38	540	35	19	10	47	10.5-13.5
Intense [3]	7.2	15.95	490	35	19	10	40	10.0-12.0

* The lower values are used with high proportion of concentrate in the diet and the higher with hay-based diet

** DM: dry matter

[1] These recommendations are suggested for geldings and mares.0.4 UFC or 0.88 Mcal NE and 30 g MADC are added daily for stallions

[2] We considered two hours of daily work (mean observed in riding school)

[3] We considered one hour of daily work

[4] For short outside riding, very light and light work intensities are considered for one and two hours of exercise, respectively. For medium (2 to 4 hours) and long (> 4 hours) outside riding, light and moderate work intensities are considered

Table 6. Requirement for growth (from Martin-Rosset et al., 1994).

Energy: relationship between daily energy intake and live weight and growth in young horses of light breeds
$UFC/day/kgW^{.75} = a+bG^{1.4}$

Ages (months)	a [1]	b
6-2	0.0602	0.0183
18-24	0.0594	0.0252
30-36	0.0594	0.0252

Protein: relationship between daily protein intake and live weight and growth in young horses of light breeds
$g\ MADC/day = aW^{.75} + bG$

Ages (months)	a [1]	b
6-12	3.5	450
12-24	2.8	270
30-36	2.8	270

[1]a: Coefficient of maintenance

G: average daily gain (kg/day)

1.4. Allometric coefficient of lipids in total body weight relatively to empty body weight

Data from Agabriel et al., 1984 & INRA unpublished results

Table 7. Energy or nitrogen requirements (500 kg BW horse) expressed either in DE and CP systems (NRC 1989) or in NE (or UFC) and MADC systems (INRA, 1984-1990) related to maintenance in each system.

Systems	Energy			Nitrogen		
Animal	NRC	INRA	% NRC/INRA	NRC	INRA	%NRC/INRA
Mature horse						
• maintenance	100	100	100	100	100	100
Growing horse						
• yearling (12 months)						
– rapid growth	130	130	100	146	227	64
– moderate growth	115	107	107	130	169	76
• 2 years old (24 months) (not in training)						
– rapid growth	148	161	92	157	156	100
– moderate growth	113	142	80	120	122	98
Working horse						
• very light	125	128	98	125	137	91
• light	-	163	-	-	174	-
• moderate	150	187	80	150	200	75
• ± intense	200	242	83	200	232	86

4. Formulating rations to meet the requirements

Formulating rations consists in choosing the feeds and determining the amounts of feeds to be offered to horses to provide them with the appropriate quantities of nutrients to meet their requirements and maintain them in good condition.

In the INRA systems the calculation of rations is very easy and has been extensively described in a handbook (INRA, 1990). Nutrient requirements and allowances can be easily determined either from tables or calculated using a software (CHEVALration) according to body weight, physiological status, and level of performance desired. Ingestibility and nutritive value of feeds and intake capacity of horses stated from experimental data by INRA are provided in feeding tables (INRA, 1990) to calculate the appropriate amounts and proportions of forages and concentrates to be used to meet the requirements. Rations can be formulated using either a graphical method or a software (CHEVALration). A method of estimation of body condition score stated from work carried out on body composition by INRA (Martin-Rosset in progress) is used to check the relevance of rationning.(INRA HN IE, 1998)

4.1 Meeting energy requirements

Meeting the energy requirements of horses depends on: 1) the intake capacity of horses expressed in kg TDMI /100Kg BW, and 2) the energy concentration of the diet offered. In the INRA system daily TDMIs determined by INRA are proposed in the tables of recommended allowances for horses at maintenance, at work or growing, according to BW. In the NRC system ranges of intake capacity are provided for horses in these situations. The energy concentration of the diet results from the nutritive value of the feeds used and the forage/concentrate ratio stated for horses in the different situations. It can be calclulated from the ratio between the daily UFC or DE requirements and TDMI provided in the tables of recommanded allowances in the INRA or NRC systems, respectively.

4.1.1 Adult horses

In the INRA system, the energy requirements of working horses (from rest to intense work) are met when the TDMI rises from 1.6 to 2.4 or 2.6 kg /100 kg BW (e.g. + 34 to 38%) and energy concentration of the diet increases from 0.54 to 0.65- 0.75 UFC/kg (e.g. + 17 to 28%). In the NRC system, for the same activities, the recommended digestible energy concentration in the diet increases from 8.4 to 12.0 MJ DE /kg TDMI (e.g. + 30%) and TDMI rises from 1.8 to 2.5 kg TDMI/100 kg BW (e.g. + 28%).

4.1.2 Young horses

The INRA recommendations for one to two-year-old horses without work range from 0.68 to 0.82 UFC/kg TDMI e.g. + 18% while TDMI increases from 1.8 to 2.1 kg/100 kg BW (e.g. + 17%) (INRA, 1990 and table 8).

The NRC recommendations for formulating diets range from: 10.4 to 8.34 MJ DE/kg TDMI, for one to 2 year-old horses not exercising e.g. + 25 p.100 for TDMI range 2.1 to 2.5 kg TDMI/100 kg BW (e.g. + 19%).

In the INRA system the energy concentration of diets for *non exercised yearlings* (320 kg BW) would be 0.82 UFC/kg TDMI because their intake capacity is limited to 2.1 kg TDMI/100 kg BW.

In *weanlings* (250 kg BW) the energy concentration of the diet should be 1 UFC/kg since TDMI is limited to 2.4 kg /100 kg BW.

In the *nursing foal*, the amount of milk and gross energy intakes per kg of daily gain (estimated by the dilution deuterium oxide as a marker of foal body water and chemical analysis of milk, respectively) are 10.6 kg and 24.4 MJ at one month of age, and 13.7 kg and 27.3 MJ at two months

Table 8. Feeding standards for the growing horses. Recommended nutrient allowances - Horses of light breed - 500 kg mature body weight (INRA 1990).

Age (months)	Mean body weight during the period (kg)	Growth		Daily allowances							Daily Feed* kg/DM**
		Level	Daily gain (g/d)	UFC	NE (Mcal)	MADC (g)	Ca (g)	P (g)	Mg (g)	Na (g)	
Yearling											
(8-12)	320	Optimal	700-800	5.5	12.10	590	39	22	10	12	5.5-8.0
	280	Moderate	400-500	4.5	9.90	440	28	16	9	9	5.0-7.5
2 year old											
(20-24)	470	Optimal	400-500	6.8	14.96	420	36	20	10	13	7.5-10.0
	440	Moderate	150-200	6.0	13.20	330	28	16	9	12	7.0-10.0
3 year old											
(32-36)	490	Optimal	150-250	6.5	14.30	330	30	18	10	12	8.0-11.0
	470	Moderate	0-100	6.0	13.20	260	25	15	8	12	7.5-10.0

* The lower values are used with high proportion of concentrates in the diet and the higher values with hay based diet

** DM: Dry Matter

of age (figures 7 and 8). Thereafter growth rate depends on both grass intake and concentrate supplementation.

4.1.3 Comparison of recommended allowances in the UFC (INRA) system and DE (NRC) system for formulating rations

The aim of any feeding system is to meet the requirement of the animals for type and level of production using available feeds. The nature, chemical composition and nutritive value of these feeds may vary with climatic and economic conditions. Ingestibility and palatability of feeds, intake capacity of animals and substitution rate between forages and concentrates must also be considered. The energy requirements (expressed in DE) of growing and working horses in the INRA and in the NRC systems have been compared by Cuddeford (1997) using conversion factors of NE to DE drawn from the INRA feed evaluation system (see above). They are slightly higher in the NRC system than in the INRA system, namely for growth.

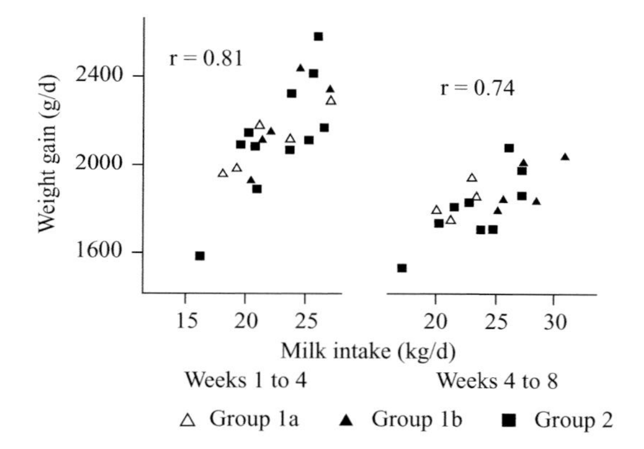

Figure 7. Relationship between foal milk intake and foal liveweight gain (from Doreau et al., 1986).

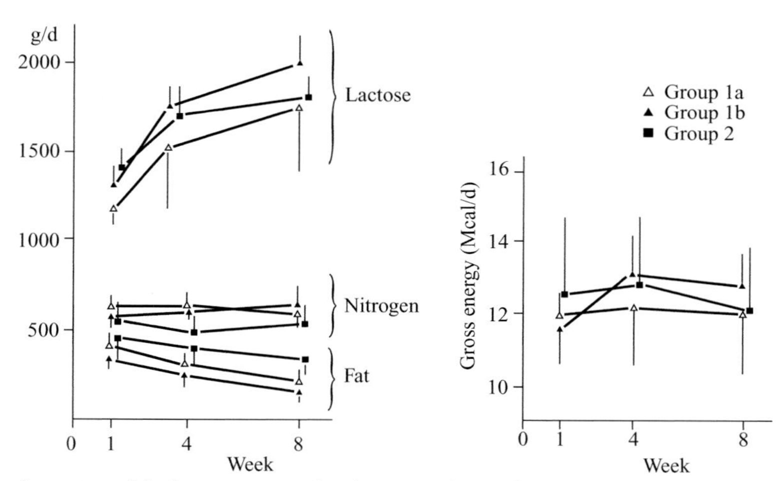

Figure 8. Quantity of foal nutrient intake (mean and standard deviation) (from Doreau et al., 1986).

However, since the nutrient requirements as well as the nutritive value of feeds and rations vary among feeding systems, it is essential to evaluate whether total energy requirements of the different types of equines can be met by the same amount of feeds in balanced rations with the various feeding systems, namely the NRC and the INRA systems.

Frape (1998) compared applications of the DE (NRC, 1989) and UFC (INRA, 1990) systems for the formulation of simple balanced daily rations based on grass hay, barley grain and extracted soyabean meal for a 500 kg mature horse.Energy and protein requirements were those proposed in each system. Feed intakes (kg DM/day) were those provided by NRC (1978). Total dry matter intakes (TDMI) for each type of animals were stated to be the same in the two feeding systems for given type of animals. As a result, the hay to concentrate ratios varied to match the energy and protein requirements in each system.

The forage dry matter intake (DMIF) is lower with the NRC system for all types of equines, except for exercising horses where it is higher. The discrepancies range from - 9 to - 24% for breeding horses and + 9 to + 19% for exercising equines. The inconsistency of the differences between the NRC and the INRA systems may partially be due to differences in energy requirements between the NRC and the INRA systems. Descriptions of, and as a result requirements for high and moderate work are different between the two systems (Martin-Rosset et al., 1994). For example, recommendations for light work in the NRC system correspond to the INRA (1990) recommendations for very light work.

Consequently, the difference between NRC and INRA systems would be greater then mentioned by Hintz and Cymbaluk (1994). The appropriate procedure to compare the two systems should be to calculate the quantities of feeds and the composition of diets necessary to meet the energy requirements of each type of equines predicted in each system according to theperformance level (DE, CP and TDMI for NRC (1989) and NE, MADC and TDMI for INRA (1990).

Good and poor (in some situations) quality hay-based diets were tested. Forages were supplemented with barley and extracted soybean meal in appropriate proportions to meet the energy and protein requirements of the different types of equines depending on their performance level. The characteristics of the four feeds used are given in table 9.

The energy value (DE or NE per kg DM) and nitrogen value (CP or MADC per kg DM) of each diet and the amount of feed required to meet energy and nitrogen requirements were computed in each energy and nitrogen system. In a first step, the hay to concentrate ratio was that proposed by

Table 9. Chemical composition and nutritive value of feeds (for NRC/INRA systems comparison).

Feeds	DM g/kg	/kg DM							
		DE (Mcal)	NE (Mcal)	CF (g)	CP (g)	DCP (g)	MADC (g)	CP/DE	MADC/NE
Good grass hay (n° 62)*	850	2.34	1.34	333	102	59	50	44	37
Poor grass hay (n° 70)*	850	1.69	0.92	382	76	37	31	45	34
Barley grain (n° 120)*	860	3.56	2.55	54	117	92	92	33	36
Soyabean meal extracted 48-50 (N° 130)*	883	4.20	2.40	39	545	496	496	130	207

* Tables INRA 1984

NRC (1989). Then, in a second step, the hay to concentrate ratio tested was that proposed by INRA (1990).

For *yearlings* (12 months old) fed good hay supplemented with the concentrate percentage proposed by the NRC, TDMI differences between the NRC and the INRA balanced rations are erratic, +/- 4 to 19% for rapid (0.750 kg/d) and moderate growth (0.450 kg /d). However, DE provided by a balanced good hay and concentrate ration calculated in the INRA system is 5 to 16% lower than DE requirements for moderate and rapid growth, respectively, in the NRC system. Conversely, the NE provided by a balance diet calculated in the NRC system is 8 to 19% higher than INRA requirements for moderate and rapid growth, respectively (see example for rapid growth in table 10). The proportion of 60% concentrate in the diet for moderate growth suggested by the NRCsystem appears to high in the INRA system; 40% would be more appropriate.

For *two -year-old* (24 months) horses not in training, fed good quality hay with 35% concentrate as proposed by the NRC, TDMI differences are erratic, +/ - 6% between NRC and the INRA systems depending on growth rate (+ 6% with the INRA ration for 0.2 kg BW gain/d and - 6% for 0.45 kg BW gain/d). But DE provided by a balanced ration calculated in the INRA system is lower (- 4%) than DE requirement according to the NRC system for rapid growth. Furthermore, NE provided by a balanced ration calculated in the NRC system is 5% higher for rapid growth and - 5% for moderate growth.

Table 10. Comparison of rations calculated in each NRC and INRA sytems balanced for energy and protein for the growing horse.

	Yearling 12 months, Rapid growth 0.750 kg/d, BW = 320 kg					
		DM (kg)	C (%)	DE (Mcal)	CP (g)	NE (Mcal)
NRC	Hay (good)	2.80		6.55	286	3.75
	Barley	3.54		12.60	414	9.03
	Soyabean	0.66	60	2.77	359	1.58
NRC Requirements		7.00		21.92	1059	14.36
21.7 Mcal DE						
1083 g CP	(2.2% BW)		NE provided by NRC ration			
2.0 < TDMI % BW <3.0						= + 2.26 Mcal
			NE requirements INRA			(+ 19%)
		DM (kg)	C (%)	NE (Mcal)	MADC (g)	DE (Mcal)
INRA	Hay (good)	2.39		3.20	120	5.59
	Barley	3.12		7.96	287	11.10
	Soyabean	0.39	60	0.93	193	1.64
INRA requirements		5.90		12.82	600	18.33
12.1 Mcal NE						
590 g MADC	(1.8% BW)		DE provided by INRAtion			
1.7 <TDMI % BW<2.5						= - 3.37 Mcal
			DE requirements NRC			(- 16%)

The interpretation of these discrepancies is confusing because of differences between the NRC and INRA requirements and interaction effects between forages and concentrates. The NRC requirements are lower than INRA requirements (table 7). The hay to concentrate ratios based on TDMI % BW suggested by NRC (1989) are rather high and very close to the maximum feed intake capacity of the growing horses fed hay ad libitum supplemented with a very high percentage of concentrate.

The forage-concentrate substitution (on a DM basis) is well known in growing horses and taken into account in the INRA system (figure 9). Forage intake decreases in the yearlings (12 months) when the amount of concentrate rises in the diet. The decreasing amount of forage DM intake, so-called substitution rate, is on average 1.26 with hays (for NE values ranging from 4.79 to 5.63 MJ /kg DM) but it is only 0.65 to 0.81 for maize silage (7.48 - 7.85 MJ NE/kg DM). Furthermore, the substitution effect might increase with age in growing horses (Martin-Rosset and Doreau, 1984b. Consequently, it is easier to understand why energy requirements of yearlings are easily met by the rations calculated in the NRC system because 1) the substitution effect is not taken into account; 2) the intake capacity stated in the NRC system is higher than in the INRA system (2.0 to 3.0 kg DM /100kg BW vs 1.7 to 2.5 kg DM/ 100kg BW). Furthermore substitution effect is still greater when the diet composition is caculated on an energy basis due to greater differences in energy value between forages and concentrates in the INRA system than in the NRC sytem. As a result, the high proportion of concentrate (35%) suggested by NRC seems overstimated for 2 year- old horses.

For *working horses*, direct comparisons are not possible since the definitions of the work intensities are different. As a result, requirements are different (table 7 and figure 6). After tentative adjustments of INRA work intensities and requirements to NRC proposals, comparisons were attempted with good hay-based diets supplemented with the percentage of concentrate proposed by the NRC system. TDMI was higher with the NRC rations than with INRA rations, regardless

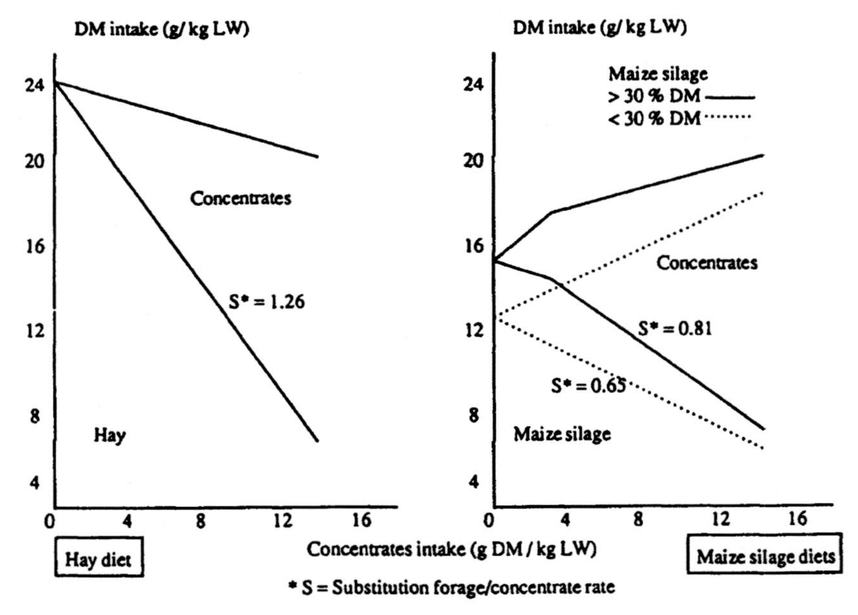

Figure 9. Effect of concentrate supplementation on forage and diet intake in young horses: 12 months of age (adapted from Agabriel et al., 1982, Martin-Rosset and Doreau 1984b).

of work intensity, and the percentages of concentrates in the NRC rations were much higher than in the INRA system. However, DE provided by the INRA rations was 12 to 18% lower than DE requirements in the NRC system.

The rations were recalculated in each system with a good hay diet supplemented with a lower percentage of concentrate and addition of some wheat straw to fit the MADC requirements in the INRA ration. TDMI was 2 to 19% higher for INRA rations than for NRC rations.

4.1.4 Validity of the energy systems

Agreements or differences in feed allowances among systems, even with the same feeds and diets, do not allow conclusions to be drawn about the validity and accuracy of each system. Animals respond to inadequate rations through changes in production (weight gain or performance), body weight and body composition.

In France, the validity of the UFC system was evaluated using two sets of data:

1. feeding trials performed at INRA with different diets based on hay (Agabriel et al., 1982; Agabriel et al., 1984; Vermorel et al., 1984; Martin-Rosset and Doreau, 1984b; Bigot et al., 1987; Martin-Rosset et al., 1989; Martin-Rosset and Vermorel, 1991; Micol and Martin-Rosset, 1995), hay, maize silage, hay-straw and supplemented with concentrates containing cereals, soyabean meal, dehy-alfalfa and bran according to type of animal (mares, growing horses, exercising horses). In addition
2. feeding experiments carried out with 8O sports horses (Selle Français and Anglo Arabe) at the National Riding School (e.g. ENE in French) settled in Saumur, and with 24 sports horses (Selle Français and Anglo Arabe) of the Equine section at the Animal Technology Teaching Centre located in Rambouillet (Vermorel et al., 1984; Martin-Rosset et al., 1989).

4.2 Metabolism and utilization of energy sources at rest and work

4.2.1 Body reserves

Free energy (e.g. ATP) required to supply energy expenditure is provided by mobilisation and catabolism of glycogen as a glucose source and triglycerides as glycerol and long chain fatty sources.

Glycogen reserves are located mainly in muscles and in the liver. In the performance horse at rest glycogen content may vary from one muscle to the other. Glycogen reserves can be increased by training (Goodmann et al., 1973; Lindholm and Piehl, 1974; Guy and Snow, 1977) but to a lesser extent than in human. In a 500 kg BW trained horse at rest the glycogen reserve ranges from 4.5 to 5.5 kg, which is very low compared to the 80 - 85 kg of adipose tissues (Martin-Rosset, 2001). Lipids reserves may provide 36 to 38 times more potential energy than the glycogen reserves.

4.2.2 Utilisation of energy sources at rest and work

At rest or for short light exercicse at walk pace, non esterified fatty acids (NEFA) and acetate are the major energy sources (Goodmann et al., 1973), whereas glucose provides only 9 to 16% of energy depending on the proportion of cereals in the diet (Argenzio et Hintz, 1972). The respiratory quotient (RQ) is below 0.9 (figure 10).

During *short and moderate exercices* at a velocity lower than 300 m/min, the oxidative catabolism of plasma glucose and NEFA and intra muscular glycogen and lipids increases. The contribution of lipids rises very quickly as shown by the reduction of the RQ to 0.8 (figure 10).

a

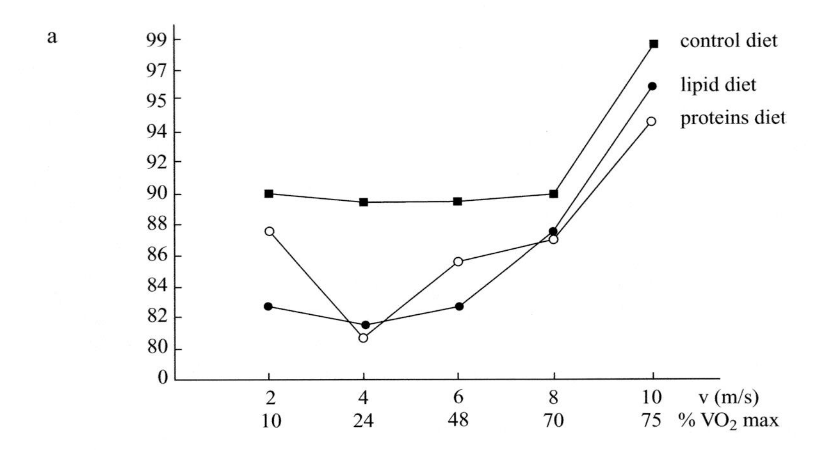

b

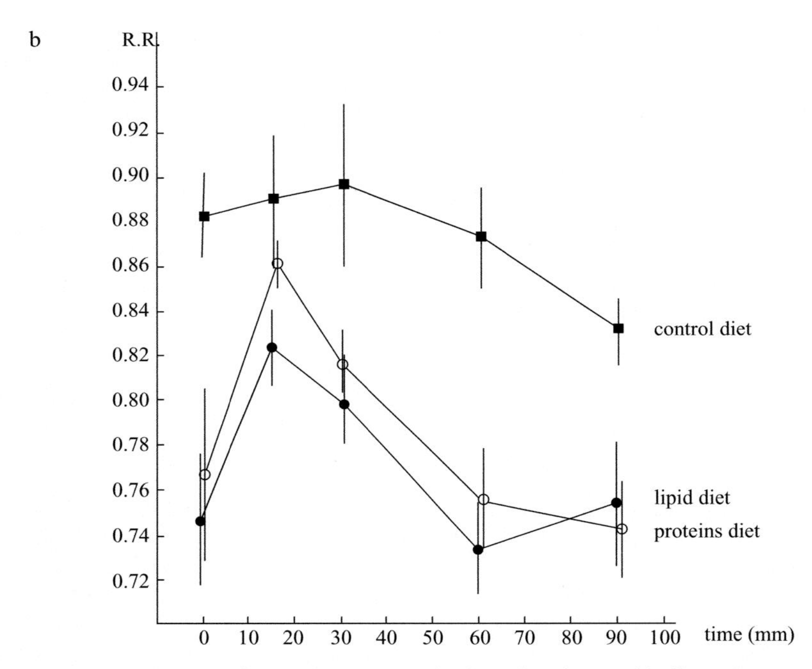

Figure 10. a. Variation of respiratory rate (RR) with velocity (v) (from Pagan et al., 1991). b. Variation of respiratory rate (RR) with duration at trot 300 m/mn (from Pagan and Hintz 1991).

During *long exercise at moderate intensity* (e.g. endurance trials: 40 to 160 km run at 12-18 km/h) the oxydative catabolism still predominates (figure 10). The contribution of lipids to energy supply increases up to reach 10 times that of glycogen (Lindholm, 1979), while plasma lactate and ketone bodies concentrations remain low.

At velocities above 300-400 m/min for trot and probably more for gallop, corresponding to 50% of V02 max, muscle fast twicht (FT) fibres are mobilized. The contribution of muscle glycogen to energy supply becomes predominant and muscular lactate content rises exponentially (Kryzwanek et al., 1972; Engelhart et al., 1973; Lindholm and Saltin, 1974; Wilson et al., 1983). As a result carbohydrates are of major concern in energy metabolism of exercising horses.

4.2.3 Response to conditionning and recovery

Two situations should be considered either for conditionning and recovery: *high intensity exercise* and *long term submaximal exercise.*

For *high intensity exercise* training aim at improving acceleration capacity of horses, elevating the fatigue threshold occurrence due the to lactate accumulation in the muscle by hypertrophia of muscular fibres, and elevation of the anaerobic threshold (cf. Review of Snow, 1983). The last physiological point is reached if several conditions are met: 1) increase in oxygen supply and captation by muscles, 2) maximum utilisation of NEFA by muscles, 3) rise in the activity of the enzymes involved in the oxidative metabolism.

Training can increase the contribution of fat to energy supply during exercise as it has been pointed out by Gollnick (1985): the RQ is lower and the rate of glycogen utilization is reduced in trained horses during exercise. In horses as in humans and dogs, training could also stimulate the ability to utilize intra muscular triglycerides during exercise while the catecholamine response would be reduced and plasma NEFA would be lowered (Issekutz and Paul, 1968; Hurtley et al., 1986; Holloszy, 1990).

After a high intensity exercise, the plasma lactate concentration decreases within a few minutes. Lactate is used for glycogen resynthesis or for oxydation in the liver and muscles(Lindinger et al., 1990). Plasma glucose concentration increases (Snow et al., 1983) probably because hepatic glycogenolysis and gluconeogenesis increase. Plasma NEFA concentration may not rise immediately after exercice because there may be still some uptake (Snow et al., 1983). But mobilization of fatty acids from adipose tissues occurs during the recovery period because glycerol concentration elevates 10 folds (Harris et al., 1987).

Long term submaximal exercise training aims at increasing first endurance of horses then velocity (e.g. in metabolic terms, to improve utilization of plasma NEFA to spare glycogen), delay the occurrence of fatigue due to the lack of glycogen and finally to elevate the anaerobic threshold where lactate accumulates. From data obtained in the marathonian humans it could be assumed than in horses the greatest part of energy is provided from lipids metabolism. The increase in plasma NEFA concentration improves their utilization and reduces the captation and utilization of glycogen by muscles (Wilmore and Freund Beau, 1980), In well trained horses, plasma NEFA concentrations are increased (Hambleton et al., 1980), plasma glucose concentration is higher, whereas plasma lactate and cortisol concentrations are lower (Grosspkopf et al., 1983).

During recovery plasma lactate is low, glucose concentration is often depressed, carbohydrates stores are deeply reduced (Lindholm and Saltin, 1974). If no extra carbohydrate are offered, glycogen repletion will rely on glycogeneogenis. Insulin concentration is low while levels of glucagon, cortisol and catecholamines are elevated and stimulate mobilization of fatty acids and glycerol.

For both types of exercises, consumption of carbohydrates is necessary to replete muscle and liver glycogen stores. The amount and timing of carbohydrate supply are of major concern to control the rate of glycogen repletion. Fom the results of human studies the best strategy for a quick repletion of glycogen stores would be the consumption of carbohydrates from 6 to 24 hours after exercise at 2 hours intervals (Costill and Hargreaves, 1992; Friedman et al., 1991). Conversely, increase in glycogen content of muscles (Kline and Albert, 1981) by offering incremental proportions of starch in the diet before exercise is much more limited in horses than in human athletes (Wilmore and Freund Beau, 1984).

Enrichement of diet with fat (7 to 16%) would stimulate the activity of the enzymes involved in lipid catabolism to promote the utilization of lipid stores, as pointed out by the depression of plasma glucose concentration (Hambleton et al., 1980; Hintz, 1983) and the improvement of performance in endurance horses (Slade et al., 1975).

4.3 Choice of feed energy sources

Cereals are obviously of major concern to feed exercising horses. However, should oat be preferred to other grains? Comparing corn and oat offered to polo horses at the same level of DE intake did not show any significatant difference in the performance of horses (Hintz, 1982). This supports the results of previous works of Wolff et al., (1888-1895), and Grandeau et al. (1904) carried out with draught horses in Europe. The negative effect of corn pointed out by horsemen is likely due to errors in formulating diets, using volume instead of weight or energy value of grains. Indeed, it is well known that one litre of corn provides 50% more NE than one litre of oat. In addition, since the MADC / UFC ratio of cereals is as high as that of forages, formulating diets with high proportions of cereals supplies horses with excess protein, which could reduce the performance (cf. Martin-Rosset and Tisserand's report in this issue).

Fat might be an alternative as it has been tested namely for endurance horse (Slade et al., 1975; Hintz, 1968 and 1983; Wolter and Valette, 1985). The NE content of 1 kg DM of fat is 2.5 fold higher than that of 1 kg of grains. Fat included in compound feeds is well accepted by horses (Bowman et al., 1977; Hintz et al., 1978; Kane et al., 1979; Rich et al., 1981; Wolter and Valette, 1985; Potter et al., 1992). Energy digestibility of vegetable fat (85 to 95%) is higher than that of animals fat (75 to 85%).

The other key-question claimed by horsemen is the following: is there any energy source to be fed to increase the available energy reserve for intensive work?

Glycogen reserves cannot be elevated in horse as high as in humans. Muscular glycogen content rises when the starch content of thediet increases from 1.9 to 2.3 and 2.5% for diets without starch, with 50% oat or enriched with 35% corn starch, respectively (Kline and Albert 1981). In addition, plasma glucose and NEFA concentrations in horses moderately exerciced are not significantly modified (Topliff et al., 1987). But increased utilization of glucose for short and intense exercice is associated with high production of lactate as shown by the linear relationship between the of muscular glycogen content and plasma lactate concentration (Pagan et al., 1987).

Dehydrated beet pulp might be a partial alternative to grains in diets of working horses to reduce excess of nitrogen intake due both to a high proportion of grains in the diet and to the high MADC/UFC ratios of grains and forages (ref. to Martin-Rosset and Tisserand's report in this issue). Dehydrated beet pulp is a highly fermentable fibre source, poor in nitrogen but with a satsifactory energy value (0.79 UFC e.g.7.30 MJ NE/kg) compared to grain (barley: 1.16 UFC e.g. 9.42 MJ/Kg).

Substituing 15% of DE of grains for dehydrated beet pulp had a similar effect on horses performing an intense exercice on a treadmill, evaluated with different plasma criteria (lactate, glucose, cortisol, insuline and triglycerydes) (Crandell et al., 2001).

5. Conclusion

The interest of the INRA system is justified by the differences in methane and urinary losses and in the effeciency of digestion end products utilisation, which induce great variations in the efficency of ME utilization. The validity of the system has been extensively tested at INRA with digestion and energy balance studies. Consequently, the energy value of feedstuffs is more accurately estimated and predicted in the INRA system than in the NRC system.

Energy requirements and recommended allowances stated in the INRA system are consistent for growing and exercising horses since they have been extensively validated using long term feeding trials. Energy requirements of horses are in most cases lower than those proposed in the NRC system.However, the allowances for intense exercice in the adult and in the 2 year- old horses, and the effect of intense exercice on lean body mass growth have to be refined in the next future, whatever the system. The last point should be studied in connection with the protein requirements (ref. to Martin-Rosset and Tisserand's report in this issue).

The utilization of the various sources of energy for long term feeding of horses (weeks) as well as the strategy to use them for short term feeding (before, during and after the competition event) have to be studied in interaction with the variation of body reserves when a training programme is accurately designed.

References

Agabriel, J., Trillaud-Geyl, C., Martin-Rosset, W. and Jussiaux, M., 1982. Utilisation de l'ensilage de maïs par le poulain de boucherie. Bull. Techn. CRZV Theix, INRA, 49: 5-13.

Agabriel, J., Martin-Rosset, W. and Robelin, J., 1984. Croissance et besoins du poulain. Chapitre 22. In: R. Jarrige, W. Martin-Rosset Editor «Le cheval» INRA Publications, route de St Cyr, 78000 Versailles. P. 370-384.

Anderson, C.E., Potter, G.D., Kreider, J.L. and Courtney, C.C., 1983. Digestible energy requirements for exercising horses. J. Anim. Sci., 41: 568-571.

Andrieu, J. and Martin-Rosset, W., 1995. Chemical, biological and physical (NIRS) methods for predicting organic matter digestibility of forages in horse. *Proceedings 14th Equine Nutrition and Physiology Symp.*,Ontario, CA, USA, pp. 76-77.

Andrieu, J., Jestin, M. and Martin-Rosset, W., 1996. Prediction of the organic matter digestibility (OMD) of forages in horses by near infra-red spectrophotometry (NIRS). In: *Proceedings of the 47th European Association of Animal Production Meeting*. Lillehammer, Norway, August, 26-29, Abstract H 4.5, p. 299. Wageningen Pers Ed. Wageningen. The Netherlands.

Argenzio R.A. and Hintz H.F., 1972. Effects of diet on glucose entry and oxidation rates in ponies. J. Nutr. 102: 879-892

Armstrong, D.G., 1969. Cell bioenergeties and energy metabolism. In : *Handbuch der Tierernährung* Ed. W. Lenkeit, K.. Breirem et E. Crasemann, pp. 385- 414, Paul Parey Hamburg Berlin.

Austbø, D., 1996. Energy and protein evaluation systems and nutrien recommendations for horses in the Nordic countries. In: *Proceedings of the 47th European Associations of Animal Production Meeting*. Lillehammer, Norway, August, 26-29, Abstract H4.4, p. 293. Wageningen Pers Ed. Wageningen The Netherlands.

Axelsson, J., 1949. Standard for nutritional requirement of domestic animals in the Scandinavian Countries. In: Ve Congrès Int. de Zootechnie, Paris, Vol. 2, Rapports particuliers, pp. 123-144.

Bigot, G., Trillaud-Geyl, C., Jussiaux, M. and Martin-Rosset, W., 1987. Elevage du cheval de selle du sevrage au débourrage: Alimentation hivernale, croissance et développement. Bul. Tech. Theix INRA. 69: 45-53.

Bowman, V.A., Fontenot, J.P., Meacham, T.N. and Webb, K.E. JR., 1979. Acceptability and digestibility of animal vegetable and blended fats by equine. In Proc. 6th Equine Nutr. Physiol. Symp. Texas AM University, 17-19

Breuer, L.H.,1968. Energy nutrition of the light horse. Proc. 1st Eq. Nutr. Res. Symp., 8-9.

Brody, S., 1945. Bioenergetics and growth. Hafner Pub. Co. New-York, 1023 pp.

Costill, D.L. and Hargreaves, M., 1992. Carbohydrate nutrition and fatigue. Sports Med. 13 (2) 86

Crandell, K., Pagan, J.D., Harris, P. and Duren, S.E., 2001. A comparison of grain, vegetable oil and beet pulp as energy sources for the exercised horse. In Advances on Equine Nutrition II. Ed. J.D. Pagan and R.J. Geor. Nottingham Press University Nottingham UK, p. 487

Cudderford, D., 1997. Feeding systems for horses. Chap. 11. In: Feeding systems and feed evaluation models. Theodorou, M.K., France J., Ed. Cabi Publishing, Oxon, U.K., NY, USA, p. 239-274.

Cymbaluck, N.F. and Christison, G.L., 1990. Environmental effects on thermoregulation and nutrion of horses. Veterinary Clinics of North America. Equine Practice 6. 355-372

Doherty, O., Booth, M., Waran, N., Salthouse, C. and Cuddeford, D., 1997. Study of the heart rate and energy expenditure of ponies duriig transport. Veterinary Record 141: 589-592

Doreau, M., 1978. Comportement alimentaire du cheval à l'écurie. Ann. Zootech. 27 (3): 291-302

Doreau, M., Boulot, S., Martin-Rosset, W., Robelin, J., 1986. Relation between nutrient intake, growth and body composition of nursing foal. Reprod. Nut. Dev., 26(B): 683-690.

Doreau, M., Martin-Rosset, W. and Boulot S., 1988. Energy requirements and the feeding of mares during lactation: a review. Livest. Prod. Sci., 20: 53-68.

Engelhardt, W.V., Hornicke, H., Ehrlein, H.I. and Schmidt, E., 1973. Lactat. Pyruvirat. Glucose and Wasserstoffionen im venösen Blut bei Reitpferden in unterschiedlichem Trainingszustamd. Zbl. Vet. Med. As. 20: 173-187

Fingerling, G., 1931-1939. quoted by Nehring K., Franke E.R., 1954

Frape, D., 1998. Equine Nutrition and Feeding. 2nd Ed. Blackwell. Science Ltd, London, pp. 564.

Friedman, J.E., Neuler, P.D. and Dohm, G.L., 1991. Regulation of glycogen re-synthesis following exercise. Sports Med. 11 (4): 232

Franke, E.R., 1954. Die Verdaulichkeit verschiedener Futtermittel beim Pferd. In 100 Jahre Möcken; Die Bewertung der Futterstoffe und andere Probleme der Tierernährung, vol. 2: 441-472

Geay, Y., Robelin, J., Beranger, C., Micol, D., Gueguen, L. and Malterre, C., 1978. Bovins en croisance et à l'engrais. In Jarrige R. (ed.) Alimentation des ruminants. INRA Publications, Versailles, France, pp. 297-344

Gollnick, P.D., 1977. Exercise, adrenergic blockage and FFA mobilization. Am. J. Phys. 213, 734-738

Goodman, H.M., Vander Noot, G.W., Trout, J.R. and Squibb, R.L., 1973. Determination of energy source utilized by the light horse. J. Anim. Sci. 37: 56-62

Grandeau, L. and Alekan, A., 1904. Vingt années d'expériences sur l'alimentation du cheval de trait. Etudes sur les rations d'entretien, de marche et de travail. Ed. L. Courtier, Paris. p. 20-48.

Grosskopf, J.F.W. and Van Rensburg, J.J., 1983. Some observations on the haematology and blood chemistry of horses compteing in 80 km endurance rides. In Equine exercise Physiology. Ed. D.H. Snow, S.G.B. Persson and R.J. Rose, 425-431, Granta Edition, Cambridge

Guy, P.S. and Snow, D.H., 1977. The effect of training and detraining on muscle composition in the horse. J. Physiol. 269: 33-51

Hambleton, P.L., Slade, L.M., Hamar, D.W., Kienholz, E.W. and Lewis, L.D., 1980. Dietary fat and exercise conditionning effect on metabolic parameters in the horse. J. Anim. Sci., 51: 1330-1339

Harris, R.C., Marlin, D.J. and Snow, D.H., 1987. Metabolic response to maximal exercise of 800 and 2000 m in the thoroughbred horse. J. Appl. Physiol., 63 (1) 12

Hintz, H.F., 1968. Energy utilization in the horse. Proc. Cornell Nutr. Conf., pp. 47-49.

Hintz, H.F., Ross, M.W., Lesser F.R., Leids, P.F., White, K.K., Lowe, J.E., Short, C.E. and Schryver, H.F., 1978. The value of dietary fat for working horses. I. Biochemical and Hematological ealuations. J. Equine Med. Surg., 2: 483.

Hintz, H.F., 1983. Nutritional requirements of the exercising horse. A review. In: *Proceedings 1st Equine exercise Physiology Symposium*, Snow D.H., Persson S.G.B., Rose R., Editors, ICEEP Publications Cambridge, p. 275-290.

Hintz, H.F. and Cymbaluk, N.F., 1994. Nutrition of the horse. Ann. Rev., 14: 243-267.

Hoffmann, L., Klippel, W. and Schiemann, R., 1967. Untersuchungen über den Energieumsatz beim Pferd unter besonderer Berücksichtigung der Horizontal bewegung. Archiv. Tierern., 17: 441-449.

Holloszy, J.O., 1990. Utilization of fatty acids during exercise. In Bio-chemistry of Exercise. Champaign, Ill, Human Kinetics Publishers, p. 319

Hörnicke, H., Ehrlein, H.J., Tolkmitt, G., Nagel, M., Epple, E., Decker, E., Kimmich, H.P. and Kreuzer, F., 1974. Method for continuous oxygen consumption measurement in exercising horses by telemetry and electronic data processing. In: *Energy metabolism of farm animals*, K.H. Menke et al., Ed. EAAP Publ. N° 14: 257-260, Stuttgart.

Hörnicke, H., Meixner, R. and Pollmann, R., 1983. Respiration in exercising horses. p.7-16. In: Equine exercice Physiology. Editors. D.H. Snow, S.G.B. Persson et R.J. Rose, Granta Edition, Cambridge.

Hurtley, B.F., Nemeth, P.M. and Martin, III WH et al., 1986. Muscle triglyceride utilization during exercise. Effect of training. J. Appl. Physiol. 60 (2): 562

INRA, 1984. Le Cheval: Reproduction, Sélection, Alimentation, Exploitation. R. Jarrige et W. Martin-Rosset Editors. INRA Edition Route de St-Cyr 78000 Versailles. pp. 689.

INRA, 1984. Tables de la valeur nutritive des aliments pour le cheval. In: R. Jarrige, W. Martin-Rosset Editors. «Le Cheval» Reproduction - Sélection - Alimentation - Exploitation. INRA Publications, Route de St Cyr, 78000 Versailles, p. 661-689.

INRA, 1984. Tables des apports alimentaires recommandés pour le cheval. In: R. Jarrige, W. Martin-Rosset Editors. «Le Cheval». INRA Publications, Route de St Cyr, 78000 Versailles, p. 645-660.

INRA, 1990. L'alimentation des chevaux. W. Martin-Rosset (Editor) INRA Publications, Route de St Cyr, 78000 Versailles. pp.232.

INRA, IE, HN, 1997. Notation de l'état corporel des chevaux de selle et de sport. Institut de l'Elevage Editions, 149 Rue de Bercy, 75595 PARIS Cedex 12, pp. 40.

Issekutz, B. Jr. and Paul, P. 1968. Intramuscular energy sources in exercising normal and pancreatectomized dogs. Am. J. Physiol. 215 (1): 197

Jespersen, J., 1949. Normes pour les besoins des animaux: chevaux, porcs et poules, in: Vème Congrès International de Zootechnie, Paris, Vol. 2, Rapports particuliers, pp. 33-43.

Kane, E., Baker, J.P. and Bull, L.S., 1979. Utilization of a corn oil supplemented diet by the pony. J. Anim. Sci. 48: 1379-1384

Karlsen, G. and Nadal'Jak, E.A., 1964. Gas-energie Umstaz une Atmung Bei Trabern Während der Arbeit. Nonevodstvo i konnyi sport, 11: 27-31.

Kellner, O., 1909. Principes fondamentaux de l'alimentation du bétail. 3ème Ed. Allemande, traduction, A. Grégoire, Berger Levrault, Paris, Nancy, pp. 288.

Kline, K.H. and Albert, W.W., 1981. Investigation of a glycogen loading programm for standarbred horses. In Proc. 7th Equine Nutr. Physio. Symp. Warenton, Virginia, p. 186-194

Kossila, V., Virtanen, R. and Maukonen, J., 1972. A diet of hay and oat as a source of energy digestible crude protein, minerals and trace elements for saddle horses. J. Sci. Agric. Soc. Finland, 44: 217-227.

Krzywanek, H., Schulze, A. and Wittke, G., 1972. Behaviour of some blood values in trotting horses after a defined work. Berliner Munchener Tierazt. Wwochenschr., 85: 325-329

Kushmerick, M.J. and Davies, R.E., 1969. The chemical energetics of muscle contraction. II. The chemistry, efficiency and power of maximally working sartorius muscles. Proc. Roy. Soc. London B, 174: 315-353

Lindholm, A. and Piehl, K., 1974. Fibre composition, enzyme activity and concentrtions of metaboliltes and electrolytes in muscles of Standardbred horses. Acta. Vet. Scand. 15: 287-309

Lindholm, A. and Saltin, B., 1974. The physiological and biochemical response of standarbred horses to exercise of varying speed and duration. Acta Vet. Scand. 15: 310-324

Lindholm, A., 1979. Substrate utilization and muscle fibre types in standardbred trotters during exercise. Proc. Am. As. Equine Pract. 25: 329-336

Lindinger, M.I., Heigenhauser, G.J.F., McKelvie, R.S. et al., 1990. Role of non-working muscle on blood metabolites and ions with intense intermittent exercise. Am. J. Physiol. 258 (Reg. Integr. Comp. Physiol.27) R1486

Livesey, G., 2001. A perspective on food energy standards for nutrition labelling. Brit. J. Nutr., 85, 271-287

McBride, G.E., Christopherson, R.J. and Sauer, W., 1985. Metabolic rate and plasma thyroïd hormone concentrations of mature horses in response to changes in ambient temperature. Canadian Journal of Animal Science 65: 375-382

Martin-Rosset, W., Boccard, R., Jussiaux, M., Robelin, J. and Trillaud-Geyl, C., 1983b. Croissance relative des différents tissus, organes et régions corporelles entre 12 et 30 mois chez le cheval de boucherie de différentes races lourdes. Ann. Zootech., 32: 153-174.

Martin-Rosset W., Andrieu J., Vermorel M. and Dulphy J.P., 1984. Valeur nutritive des aliments pour le cheval. Chapter 17. In R. Jarrige, W. Martin-Rosset Editors. «Le Cheval» INRA Publications, Route de St Cyr, 78000 Versailles, p. 208-239

Martin-Rosset W. and Doreau M., 1984b. Consommation des aliments et d'eau par le cheval. Chapter 22. In R. Jarrige, W. Martin-Rosset Editors. «Le Cheval» INRA Publications, Route de St Cyr, 78000 Versailles, p. 334-354

Martin-Rosset, W., Boccard, R., Robelin, J., Jussiaux, M., Trillaud-Geyl, C., 1985. Estimation de la composistion de la carcasse des poulains de boucherie à partir de la composition de l'épaule ou d'un morceau monocastal prélevé au niveau de la 14e côte. Ann. Zootech., 34: 77-84.

Martin-Rosset, W. and Dulphy, J.P. 1987. Digestibility. Interactions between forages and concentrates in horses': influence of feeding level. Comparison with sheep. Livest. Prod. Sci., 17: 263-276.

Martin-Rosset, W., Tavernier and Vermorel, M., 1989. Alimentation du cheval de club avec un régime à base de paille et d'aliments composés. Proceedings 15e Journée Recherche Chevaline. Paris -8 mars - CEREOPA Ed. 16 rue Claude Bernard 75231 Paris Cedex 05, p.90-102.

Martin-Rosset, W., Doreau, M. Boulot, S. and Miraglia, N., 1990..Influence of level of feeding and physiological state on diet digestibility in light and heavy breed horses. Livest. Prod. Sci., 25: 257-264.

Martin-Rosset, W. and Vermorel, M., 1991. Maintenance energy requirements determined by indirect calorimetry and feeding trials in light horses. Eq. Vet. Sci., 11: 42-45.

Martin-Rosset, W., Vermorel, M., Doreau, M., Tisserand, J.L. and Andrieu, J., 1994. The French horse feed evaluation systems and recommended allowances for energy and protein. Livest. Prod. Sci., 40: 37-56.

Martin-Rosset, W., Andrieu, J. and Vermorel, M., 1996a. Routine methods for predicting the net energy value (UFC) of feeds in horses. In: Proceedings 47th European Association for Animal Production Meeting, Lillehammer, Norway, August, 26-29, Horse Commission. Session IV. Abstract H 4.1. p. 292. Wageningen Pers Ed. Wageningen The Netherlands (full paper, pp. 14).

Martin-Rosset, W., Andrieu, J. and Jestin, M., 1996b. Prediction of the digestibility of organic matter of forages in horses from the chemical composition. In: Proceedings of the 47th European Association of Animal Production Meeting. Lillehammer, NorNay, August, 26-29, Abstract H4.7, p. 295. Wageningen Pers Ed. Wageningen The Netherlands (full paper, pp. 6).

Martin-Rosset, W., Andrieu, J. and Jestin, M., 1996c. Prediction of the digestibility of organic matter of forages in horses by pepsin-cellulase method. In: *Proceedings of the 47th European Association of Animal Production Meeting*. Lillehammer, Norway, August, 26-29, Abstract H4.6, p.294. Wageningen Pers Ed. Wageningen The Netherlands (full paper, pp. 6).

Martin-Rosset, W., 2001. Feeding standards for energy and protein for horses in France. In Advances in Equine Nutrition II, J.D. Pagan and R.J. Geor Ed. Ker, Nottingham University Press, p. 245-305.

Meixner, R., Hörnicke, H. and Ehrlein, H.J., 1981. Oxygen consumption, pulmonary ventilation and heart rate of riding-horses during walk, trot and gallop. Biotelemetry, p.6.

Micol, D. and Martin-Rosset, W., 1995. Feeding systems for horses on high forage diets in the temperate zones. Chapter 15. In: *Proceedings IVth International Symposium Nutrition Herbivores*. M. Journet et al., Editors Clermont-Ferrand. September 11-15, INRA Edition Route de St-Cyr 78000 Versailles, p.569-584.

Miraglia, N. and Olivieri, O., 1990. Statement and expression of the energy and nitrogen value of feedstuffs in Southern Europe In: *Proceedings of the 41st European Association of Animal Production Meeting*. Toulouse, France, Abstract p. 390. Wageningen Pers. Ed. The Netherlands.

Nadal'Jak, E.A., 1961. Gaseous exchange in horses in transport work at the walk and trot with differents loads and rates of movements. Gaseous exchange and energy expenditure at rest and during different tasks by breeding stallions of heavy draught breeds. Effect of state of training on gaseous exchange and energy expendure in horses of heavy draught breeds (in russian). Nutr. Abstr. Reviews, 32, n° 2230-2231-2232: 463-464.

Nehring, K., Franke, E.R., 1954. Untersuchungen über den Stoff und Energieumsatz und den Nährwert verschiedener >Futtermittel beim Pferd. In : Untersuchungen über die Vewertung von reinen Nährstoffen und Futterstoffer mit Hilfe von Restpirationsversuchen. K. Nehring, vol. 3: 255-358. Deutsche Akademic Berlin.

NRC, 1978. Nutrient requirements of domestic animals. n° 6. Nutrient Requirements of Horses, 4th revised edition. National Academy of Sciences, Washington, D., pp 33.

NRC, 1989. Nutrient requierements of horses, Rth Revised edition. Subcommittee on Horse Nutrition Board on Agriculture National Academy Press - Washington D.C., pp. 100.

Pagan, J.D. and Hintz, H.F., 1986b. Equine energetics. II. Energy expenditure in horses during submaximal exercise. *J. of Anim. Sci.*, 63: 822-830.

Pagan, J.D., Essen-Gustavsson, Lindholm, M. and Thornton, J., 1987. The effect of dietary energy source on exercise performance in standard breed horses. In: *Proceedings, 2nd exercise Physiology Symposium*, Gillepsie J.R. and Robinson N.E., Editions ICEEP Publications, Davis, USA, p. 686-701.

Rich, V.B., Fontenot, J.P. and Meacham, T.N., 1981. Digestibility of animal, vegetable and blended fats by equine. Proc. 7th Equine Nutr. Physiol. Symp. Warrenton Virginia, 30-36

Robelin, J., 1979. Influence de la vitesse de croissance sur la composition du gain de poids des bovins; variations selon la race et le sexe. Annales Zooechnie 28: 209-218

Slade, L.M., Lewis, L.D., Quinn, C.R. and Chandler, M.L., 1975. Nutritional adaptations of horses for endurance performance. Proc. Equine Nutr. Soc. 114-128

Smolders, E.A.A., 1990. Evolution of the energy and nitrogen systems used in The Netherlands. In: *Proceedings of the 41st European Association of Animal Production Meeting*. Toulouse, France, p. 386 (abstract). Wageningen Pers. Ed. Wageningen The Netherlands.

Snow, D.H., 1983. Skeletal muscle adaptations. A review. In Equine exercise physiol. Ed. D.H. Snow, S.G.B. Persson et R.J. Rose, 160-183. Granta Editio, Cambridge

Staun, H., 1990. Energy and nitrogen systems used in northern countries for estimating and expressing value of feedstuffs in horses. In: *Proceedings of the 41st European Association of Animal Production Meeting*. Toulouse, France, Abstract p. 388.Wageningen Pers. Ed. Wageningen The Netherlands.

Stillions, M.C. and Nelson, W.E., 1972. Digestible energy during maintenance of the light horse. J. Anim. Sci., 34: 981-982.

Topliff, D.R., Lee, S.F. and Freeman, D.W., 1987. Muscle glycogen, plasma glucose and free fatty acides in exercising horse fed warying levels of starch. In Proceeding 10th ENPS Colorado, USA, June 11-13th, 421-424.

Vermorel, M., Jarrige, R. and Martin-Rosset, W., 1984. Métabolisme et besoins énergétiques du cheval. Le système des UFC. Chapter 18. In: R. Jarrige et, W. Martin-Rosset (Editors). «Le Cheval» INRA Publications, Route de St Cyr, 78000 Versailles, p. 237-276.

Vermorel M. and Mormède P., 1991. Energy cost of eating in ponies. In C. Wenk and M. Boessiger (Eds.). Energy Metabolism of farm Animals. Institu für Nutztierwissenschaften. EAAP Publ. N° 58. ETH Zentrum. CH-8092 Zurih pp. 437-440

Vermorel, M., Martin-Rosset, W. and Vernet, J., 1991. Energy utilization of two diets for maintenance by horses: agreement with the new french net energy system. Eq. Vet. Sci., 11: 33-35.

Vermorel, M., Martin-Rosset, W. and Vernet, J., 1997. Energy utilization of twelve forages or mixed diets for maintenance by sport horses. Livest. Prod. 57: 157-167.

Vermorel, M. and Martin-Rosset, W., 1997. Concepts, scientific bases, structure and validation of the French horse net energy system (UFC). Livest. Prod. Sci., 47: 261-275.

Vernet, J., Vermorel, M. and Martin-Rosset, W., 1995. Energy cost of eating long hay, straw and pelleted food in sport horses. Journal of Animal Science 61: 581-588

Willard, J.C., Wolfram, S.A., Baker, J.P. and Bull, L.S., 1979. Determination of the energy requirement for work. Proc. 6th Equine Nutr. Physiol. Symp. Texas A.M. University, 33-34

Willmore, J.H. and Freund Beau J., 1984. Nutritional enchancement of athletic performance. Nur. Abs. Rev., Series A., 54: 1-16.

Wilson, R.G., Isler, R.B. and Thornton, J.R., 1983. Heart rate, lactic acid production and speed during a standardized exercise in standardbred horses. In Equine exercise physiol. Ed. D.H. Snow, S.G.B. Persson and R.J. Rose, 487-496, Granta Edition, Cambridge

Wolff, E. and Kreuzhage, C., 1895. Pferde Fütterungsversuche über Verdauuung und Arbeitsäquivalent des Futters. Landw. Jahrb., 24: 125-271.

Wolter R. and Valette J.P., 1985. Etude expérimentale de l'influence de régimes hyperlipidiques sur les aptitudes sportives d'équidés en effort d'endurance. 11e Journée étude CEREOPA, Ed. Paris, 122-136

Wooden, G.R., Know, K.L. and Wild, C.L., 1970. Energy metabolism of light horses. J. Anim. Sci., 30: 544-548.

Zuntz, N. and Hagemann, O., 1898. Untersuchungen über den Stoffwechsel des Pferdes bei Ruhe und Arbeit. Landw. Jahrb., 27, suppl. 3: 1-437.

The Dutch net energy system

Andrea D. Ellis

Research Institute for Animal Husbandry, Lelystad, The Netherlands

1. Predicting energy value of feedstuffs

"The food is by no means ready to enter directly into the composition of the tissues of the body and add to its store of potential energy, but on the contrary, a very considerable amount of energy must be expended in the separation of the indigestible matters from the digestible and in the conversion of the latter into such forms as are suitable for the uses of the living cells in the body."
(Armsby, 1903)

In 1995 the Centraal Veevoederbureau (CVB) has introduced an energy system specifically for horses, based on the French NE system. Some extensive in vivo research has been carried out at PV (Research Institute for Animal Husbandry) in the late 1980's (Smolders *et al.*, 1990). The authors compared 53 feedstuffs in horses and sheep at maintenance. The feed unit **VEP** (voeder eenheid paard - feeding unit horse) was introduced. The following steps to estimate net energy and VEP values for feed are taken and extensive feed value tables are published annually (CVB):

Step 1: Gross Energy Content

In The Netherlands one general equation is applied, to calculate GE of feeding stuffs for both horses and cattle, in order to promote uniformity at this level (CVB, 1996) (all chemical constituents in g/kg DM).

GE(kJ/kg DM) = 24.1 CP + 36.6 EE + 20.9 CF + 17.0 Nfe (- 0.63 SUG)[a]

[a] only subtracted if sugar content exceeds 80g/kg DM
(where Nfe = Nitrogen free Extract; SUG includes: all soluble carbohydrates in 40% ethanol; in glucose equivalents)
For maize silage a separate calculation is used: GE = 19456 - 19.456 Ash (in KJ/kg DS)

Step 2: Energy Digestibility - ED measured in horses (as Inra)

ED (VCGE) = 0.034 + Δ+ 0.9477 OMd ($VCOS_{Horses}$)

Δ = **- 1.1** for forages
Δ = **+1.1** for concentrates

Step 3: Calculating DE

DE content of feeds was derived in vivo where possible or by using the above equation and: ED as % of GE= DE

Organic Matter digestibility (OMd) was measured for 75 different feedstuffs **in horses** by INRA (France) and PV (The Netherlands) - In the Netherlands 11 fresh grasses, 19 hays, 5 dehydrated roughages, 2 legume seeds, 7 oilmeals and 9 compound feed were tested ***in vivo.***

OVERVIEW OF MAIN SYSTEMS FOR PREDICTION OF FEED ENERGY IN RELATION TO THE DUTCH SYSTEM

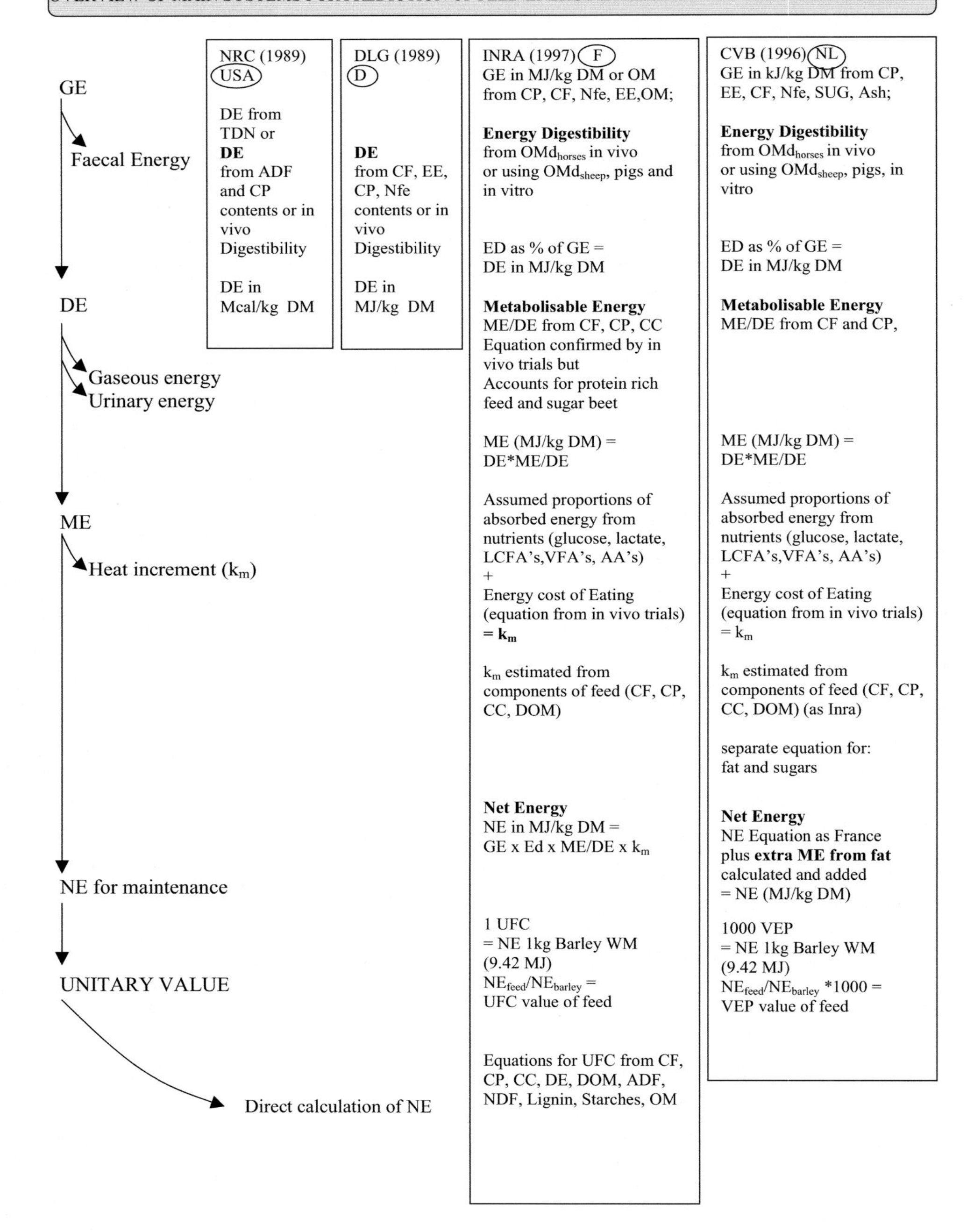

For estimation of OMd for FRESH GRASS AND HAYS ONLY, where in vivo results for horses are not available a regression co-efficient from sheep to horses has been calculated following *in vivo* research at INRA and PR - Lelystad.

$OMd_{Horses} = -16.71 + 1.1436\ OMd_{Sheep} + 4.4\ F$ (in %)
RSD = 1.8 $R^2 = 0.978$ n=27

F = 1 when using French OMd_{Sheep}
F = 0 when using Dutch OMd_{Sheep} values

Finally, if sheep data is not available the Omd_{Horses} has also been correlated for hay, fresh grasses, artificially dried forages, grass silage and individual concentrates with OMd results from the Tilley an Terry in vitro (t) digestibility method (1963):

$OMd_{Horses} = - 8.66 + 0.9712\ OMd_t + 9.07\ V$ (in %)

V = 0 for fresh grasses, hay, artificially dried forages,
V = 1 for silages and concentrates

Following comparison of OMd_{Sheep} in French and Dutch trials it was decided to add a correction for French results into the Dutch regression calculation, as French OMd_{Sheep} values lay below Dutch values (probably due to feeding levels). However, the Dutch system still predicts a 1-2% higher OMd for horses from sheep values.

Step 4: Ratio between ME and DE - determined in horses

ME (KJ/kg) = DE * ME/DE
ME/DE = (93.96 - 0.02356 CF - 0.0217 CP) / 100 $R^2 = 0.5184$ RSD = 2.02

The formula for estimating ME - DE ratio has been derived from previous research (composition in g/kg DM).

Step 5: Assumed proportions of absorbed energy supplied by various nutrients

The conversion process from ME to NE in the Dutch system is initially identical to the French system.
NE = GE x dE x ME/DE **x** $\mathbf{k_m}$

For calculation of $\mathbf{k_m}$
The formulas incorporating CF, CP and CC (Cytoplasmic Content: starch and soluble carbohydrates) from the French system have been chosen for practical application (chemical values in g/ kg DM).

	RSD	R^2
Forages:		
k_m = (65.21 - 0.01780CF + 0.0181CP + 0.0452 CC)/100	0.53	0.963
Concentrates:		
k_m = (72.34 + 0.0119CF - 0.081CP + 0.0112 CC)/100	0.35	0.990
Cereal by-products:		
k_m = (94.41-0.0237 OM - 0.0022 RE+0.0121*(STARCH + SUG))/100	0.45	0.961

Oil-production by-products:
$k_m = (67.03 - 0.004261\ RE + 0.01566*(STARCH + SUG))/100$

In the Dutch system an additional k_m value for fats (animal or plant) and for Sugar has been added, to account for extra energy derived from these:
Fat: $k_m = 0.80$ Sugar: $k_m = 0.85$

Following this the NE calculation from ME was refined to incorporate energy derived from Crude Fat (EE) in the ration. First the net energy value of EE in KJ was calculated and this was then added into the final formula:

$$ME_{EE} = GE * DE_{EE} * ME/DE_{EE} = 36.6 * 0.9 * 0.95 = 31.3\ KJ$$

$$NEm = (k_m * (ME - 31.3\ EE) + 0.80 * 31.3\ EE)/1000\ (in\ MJ)$$

If calculating the NEm value of a high-fat feed such as soya beans using either the French or Dutch Formulas 11.45 and 12.01 MJ/ kg DM are derived. Therefore the added increase by taking account of the fat values has led to a MJ increase of 0.56 compared to the French NE.

Step 6: Conversion to a 'common unit'

The common unit applied to give NE (at maintenance) values of feed is, as in the French system based on relating feed values back to barley. To comply with the VEM system the value of barley is set at 1000 VEP.

Therefore: 1kg barley is estimated at 87% DM and   GE = 16.3 MJ/kg WM
Then: DOM = 0.83   ED = 0.80   DE = 12.87 MJ/kg WM
1kg barley WM = 2250 cal = 9.414 MJ NE
1000 VEP = 9.414 MJ NE/ kg WM
1kg barley WM = 1000 VEP (1kg Barley DM = 1150 VEP)
1 VEP = 0.009414 MJ NE/kg WM

The VEP value of a feed WM (x) = NE content of feed (MJ/kg WM) /NE content of barley =

$$\frac{NE\ feed}{NE\ barley} \times 1000 \quad \text{or } VEP_{(feed)} = (NE_{feed}/9.414) \times 1000$$

Why do we use a Net Energy System in Holland for estimating feed energy for performace horses?

In order to predict the feed energy available for maintenance of weight, work or production, the NE system makes a more accurate distinction between different feed sources because it:

- incorporates a large number of in vivo OMd values (Smolders *et al.*, 1990; Martin-Rosset *et al.*, 1994)
- accounts for energy lost from urine and methane - incorporating *in vivo* research (Vermorel and Martin-Rosset, 1997)
- accounts for energy substrates derived from different feed (e.g. glucose, starches, or VFA's) - incorporating *in vitro* and *in vivo* research (Vermorel and Martin-Rosset, 1997)
- accounts for efficiency of absorption of substrates and utilisation of metabolisable energy for maintenance, depending on feed - incorporating energy cost of eating (based on *in vivo* data - Vernet *et al.*, 1995)
- Accounts for more efficient utilisation of energy derived from fats and sugar

2. Energy requirements for horses at maintenance

"Living is an expensive process. Circulation, respiration, excretion and muscle tension never cease while life remains, even under conditions of absolute rest."
(Brody, 1945)

The Dutch System uses the net energy requirements for maintenance as calculated by the French system, based on an extensive review of previous research and on in vivo trials done in France (Inra, 1984). However, the Dutch system has not taken over the distinction between riding horses and TB, but generally summarises sports horses as 'Thoroughbreds, Warmbloods and cross breeds', applying a 5% increase from basal energy for these animals. Net energy systems have different maintenance requirements according to type of horses (breed, sex), condition and work, while the DE systems operate on a basic maintenance metabolism for all horses. The energy requirements are given in the tables below for adult horses, with an example for a 500kg WB gelding (Table 1 and 2).

Table 1. Equation for daily energy requirements for horses at maintenance according to the Dutch System.

Daily requirements	kJ/kg $BW^{0.75}$		VEP / kg $BW^{0.75}$	
	Mare/Gelding	Stallion	Mare/Gelding	Stallion
Cold-blood	351	386	37	41
Warmblood,TB and x-breeds	367	404	39	43

(Source: CVB 1996)

Table 2. Mean Energy requirements in VEP for maintenance.

BW	$BW^{0.75}$	Mares and Geldings		Stallions	
kg	kg	Cold-blood horses	Warmbloods, TB and cross breeds	Cold-blood horses	Warmbloods, TB and cross breeds
100	31.6	1170	1230	1300	1360
200	53.2	1970	2070	2180	2290
300	72.1	2670	2810	2960	3100
400	89.4	3310	3490	3670	3850
500	105.7	3910	4120	4340	4550
600	121.2	4490	4730	4970	5210
700	136.1	5041	5310	5580	5850
800	150.4	5570	5870	6170	6470

Source: CVB 1996)

In order to compare differences between all systems across DE and NE the daily energy requirements need to be converted into a common unit. In this purely theoretical example straight concentrates were chosen as the common unit, as their energy content varies less between countries than forages. The energy content of maize barley and oats as per system was used to calculate daily dry matter requirements for a 600 kg riding horse (Figure 1). The NRC system for horses of this size has the highest requirements.

In terms of 'oat-units' the NRC would recommend a daily intake of 5.4 kg DM, while INRA recommends only 4.4 kg DM as sufficient to cover requirements with the other values in between. The differences occurring between the CVB and INRA system can be attributed to the adaptation of the French equations used to calculate NE of a feedstuff.

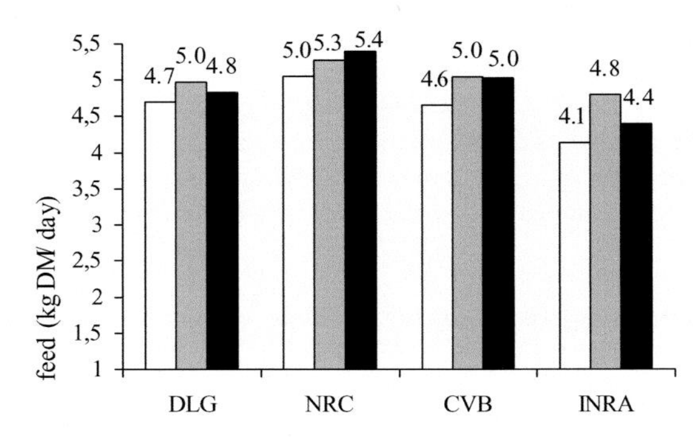

Figure 1. Daily 'feed unit' requirements for maintenance (using maize □, barley ▩ and oats ■)

Why do we base our Energy Requirements for Maintenance in Holland on the French System ?

Equations from all systems are based on several *in vivo* trials, but the general draw-back of most in vivo studies, is the low number of horses used at one set feeding level. Once an equation is set up, further *in vivo* trials need to confirm repeatability and correctness. This has occurred most extensively in the French system both for NE prediction of feedstuffs and in relation to NE requirements (Martin-Rosset and Vermorel, 1991; Vermorel *et al.*, 1997a, b).

3. Energy requirements for work

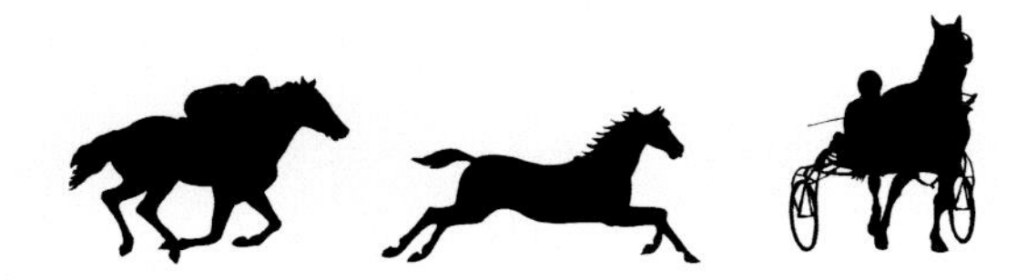

The Dutch system for evaluating energy needs of horses at work is based upon the experiments and calculations of Pagan and Hintz (1986). The efficiency of the energy metabolism for maintenance is also adjusted by 5%, i.e. the horse will need 5% more energy for maintenance if it is working (= 2 VEP/kg $LW^{0.75}$*). This is equal to the amount given in the French System for draught horses, while INRA recommends a 10% increase for the Warmblood horse and 15% for the Thoroughbred. Following this adjustment, work is then divided into light, medium and heavy work. Intensity is measured through velocity and duration of activity, thus the French system is being combined with the NE equation derived from in vivo research by Pagan and Hintz (1986). Some research into energy expenditure during exercise at PR (Smolders, 1987) confirms the calculations of Pagan and Hintz (1986) at low intensity flat work. The NE (or ME) formula is adapted to kcal/kg/min and then transformed into the Dutch feeding unit (VEP).

$Y = e^{(3.02 + 0.0065X)} - 13.92$ (in cal/ kg BW/ min)

y = Net energy in Kcal per kg BW per minute
x = speed in m/min

$VEP_{work} = ((e^{(3.02 + 0.0065X)} - 13.92) \times 4.184 \times 10^{-3}) / 9.414$ per kg (horse + rider = BW_{HR}) per min.

In the general advise table work is simply characterised by the following: walk, light, medium, heavy and very heavy. Table 3, however, gives average minutes spent within an hour to give a clearer definition of the intensity which leads to the above definitions. Velocity has been included by further sub-dividing trot and canter. For the performance horse owner this table is useful to combine changes in training times and intensity with changes in energy intake. Initially this system has very precise definitions of work, incorporating velocity, duration and weight of rider and tack. For the leisure horse owner, summary tables of energy requirements are given (Table 4):

Table 3. Characterisation of work according to intensity and duration.

	Walk	Trot	Trot	Canter	Gallop	Jumping	Total
km/hour	7	14	32	22	43	24	
m/min	120	240	540	360	720	400	
Walk	57	3	-	-	-	-	60
Light	29	29	-	2	-	-	60
Medium	14	34	-	7	-	5	60
Heavy	14	23	-	10	-	13	60
Very heavy	12	15	12	9	2	10	60

(Source: CVB 1996)

Table 4. Mean Energy Requirements in VEP for one hour work (exclusive maintenance requirements).

	Weight of horse and rider (kg)		
Work level	200 + 50	400 + 60	600 + 80
Walk	220	410	610
Light	410	760	1120
Medium	660	1220	1810
Heavy	860	1580	2340
Very heavy	2050	3780	5580

(Source: CVB 1996)

Performance horse owners are advised to increase accuracy by exact application of the above formula as suggested:

$VEP_{work} = [((e^{(3.02 + 0.0065X)} - 13.92) \times 4.184 \times 10^{-3}) / 9.414] \times kg\ BW_{HR} \times minutes$

Why have we chosen this system for working requirements ?

- The study by Pagan and Hintz (1986) is one of the most extensive studies currently available using respiratory calorimetry in modern sports horses, as a total of 304 measurements were taken.
- Our system has been set up to be used at three levels: to give general guidelines to the leisure horse owner (Table 4), allow more detailed evaluation (Table 3) or it can be used for exact calculation of energy requirements with the help of a computer program or calculator for performance horse owners, who wish to adapt feed intake regularly according to training regimes.

References

Armsby, H.P., 1903. The principles of Animal Nutrition, Chapman & Hall, London

Brody, S., 1945. Bioenergetics and Growth, Reinhold Publishing Coporation, New York

DLG, 1992. Epfehlungen zur Energie- und Nahrstoffversorgung der Pferde, DLG-Verlag, Frankfurt/Main

CVB. 1996. Documentatierrapport nr 15, Het definitieve VEP- en VREp-systeem, centraal veevoederbureau

CVB. 2000. Veevoedertabel 2000, Centraal Veevoederbureau, Lelystad

INRA. 1984. Jarrige, R. and Martin-Rosset, W. (eds.) Le Cheval, Reproduction, Selection, Alimentation, Exploitation, Instituut National de la Recherche Argronomique, Paris

Martin-Rosset, W. and Dulphy, J.P., 1987. Digestibility Interactions between Forages and Concentrates in Horses: Influence of Feeding Level - Comparison with Sheep, Livestock Production Science, 17: 263-276

Martin-Rosset, W., Doreau, M., Boulot, S. and Miraglia, N., 1990. Influence of level of feeding and physiological state on diet digestibility in light and heavy breed horses, Livestock Production Science, 25: 257-264

Martin-Rosset, W. and Vermorel, M., 1991. Maintenance energy requirements determined by indirect calorimetry and feeding trials in light horses, Equine Veterinary Science, 11: 42-45

Martin-Rosset, W., Vermorel, M., Doreau, M., Tisserand, J.L. and Andrieu, J., 1994. The French Horse Feed Evaluation System and Recommended Allowances for Energy and Protein, Livestock Production Science, 40: 37-57, INRA

Meyer, H., 1992. Pferdefütterung, 2. Auflage, Blackwell Wissenschafts-Verlag, Berlin, Wien

NRC, 1989. Nutrient Requirements of Horses, 5th ed. revised, National Academy of Sciences, Washington DC

Pagan, J.D. and Hintz, H.F., 1986. Equine Energetics. I: Relationship between body weight and energy requirements in horses, J. Anim. Sci., 63: 815-821

Vermorel, M., Martin-Rosset, W. and Vernet, J., 1997a. Energy utilisation of twelve forages or mixed diets for maintenance by sport horses, Livestock Production Sciences, 47, 157-167

Vermorel, M., Vernet, J. and Martin-Rosset, W., 1997b. Digestive and energy utilisation of two diets by ponies and horses, Livestock Production Science, 51: 13-19

Vermorel, M. and Martin-Rosset, W., 1997. Concepts, scientific basis, structure and validation of the French horse net energy system (UFC), Livestock Production Science, 47: 261-275

Vernet, J., Vermorel, M. and Martin-Rosset, W., 1995. Energy cost of eating long hay, straw and pelleted food in sport horses, Animal Science, 61: 581-588.

Smolders, E.A.A., 1987. Energy requirements during maximal exercise, EAAP, Lissabon

Smolders, E.A.A., Steg, A. and Hindle, V.A., 1990. Organic Matter Digestibility in Horses and its Prediction, Netherlands Journal of Agricultural Science, 38: 435-447

The Scandinavian adaptation of the French UFC system

Dag Austbø

Department of Animal Science, Agricultural University of Norway

The mandate of the Nordic working group "Feed evaluation and nutrient recommendations for horses" was to find a common basis for feed evaluation and nutrient recommendations in the Nordic countries (Norway, Denmark, Sweden, Finland and Island). As a result of this work, it is proposed to use the French UFC system for evaluation of energy value of feeds for horses and for calculation of energy requirements. During this work also the Dutch adaptation of the French system described in "Het definitieve VEP- en VREp-systeem", CVB-documentatierapport nr. 15, oktober 1996, was studied. The calculation of requirements for pregnancy, lactation and growth is according to the Dutch work. The French MADC system was also studied, but it was agreed not to implement this system until it had been further developed. Instead it was decided (as in Holland) to use digestible crude protein (DCP).

1. Energy

In the Nordic countries, energy is expressed as net energy (feed units) in Norway, Denmark and Island, as metabolisable energy (MJ) in Sweden and as metabolisable energy expressed as feed units in Finland (1 feed unit ME is calculated as MJ/11.7). The French UFC-system is build on data from experiments with horses, and therefore gives the opportunity to calculate energy values of feeds as digestible energy (DE), metabolisable energy (ME) or net energy (UFC). By using the UFC-system, each country could still be given the opportunity to choose how to express the energy (DE, ME or NE).

To calculate energy in the different energy units, the following factors can be used:

1 UFC (NE)	= 13.45 MJ (ME)	DK, N, Is → Sweden
1 UFC (NE)	= 1.15 F.u (ME)	DK, N, Is →(Finland
1 MJ (ME)	= 0.0743 UFC	Sweden → Denmark, Norway, Island
1 MJ (ME)	= 0.0855 F.u (ME)	Sweden → Finland
1 F.u (ME)	= 11.7 MJ (ME)	Finland → Sweden
1 F.u (ME)	= 0.87 UFC	Finland → Denmark, Norway, Island

2. Protein

Protein is expressed as digestible crude protein (DCP). Experiments have shown little difference between digestibility of crude protein for horses and sheep, and digestibility data from both species can be used without corrections. The French protein evaluation system for horses (MADC) will be considered when the system is better documented.

3. Maintenance requirement

3.1 Energy

The maintenance requirement is calculated according to metabolic body weight ($BW^{0.75}$). The calculations give requirements for cold-blooded mares and geldings.

Table 1. Calculation of the maintenance requirement for adult horses (cold-blooded).

Maint. requirement (NE)	$= 0.351$ MJ/kg $BW^{0.75}$	
Maint. requirement (NE) $= 0.351 / 9.414$	$= 0.0373$ UFC/kg $BW^{0.75}$	(DK, N, Is)
Maint. requirement (ME) $= 0.351 / 0.7$	$= 0.50$ MJ/$BW^{0.75}$	(Sweden)
Maint. requirement (ME) $= (0.351 / 0.7) / 11.7$	$= 0.0429$ ME (F.u)/$BW^{0.75}$	(Finland)

Corrections are being calculated for different types of horses (cold-blooded, warm-blooded, thoroughbred) and sex (mare/gelding, stallion).

For the Nordic countries it is suggested that the corrections for type of horse will be:

Cold-blooded ponies and draught horses	No correction
Warm-blooded horses and cold-blooded trotters	5% correction
Thoroughbred	10% correction

For stallions an extra 10% will be calculated compared to mares and geldings

Table 2. Calculation of the maintenance energy requirement for adult horses, BW 500 kg.

Country	Type of horse	Mare/Gelding	Stallion
DK, N, Is (UFC)	Cold-blooded, ponies and draught horses	3.9	4.3
	Warm-blooded horses and cold-blooded trotters	4.1	4.5
	Thoroughbred	4.3	4.7
Sweden (MJ ME)	Cold-blooded, ponies and draught horses	52.9	58.1
	Warm-blooded horses and cold-blooded trotters	55.6	61.1
	Thoroughbred	58.1	63.9
Finland (F.u ME)	Cold-blooded, ponies and draught horses	4.53	4.98
	Warm-blooded horses and cold-blooded trotters	4.76	5.24
	Thoroughbred	4.98	5.48

Horses in training have a higher maintenance requirement than horses not in training. This will be accounted for when calculating energy needs for training.

3.2 Protein

The protein requirement of adult horses is calculated as 3 g digestible crude protein (DCP) per kg $BW^{0.75}$ per day.

This is in accordance with recommendations from Germany (3.0 g per kg $BW^{0.75}$ per day), France (2.8 g per kg $BW^{0.75}$ per day) and USA (calculated mean value 2.8 g per kg $BW^{0.75}$ per day).

Table 3. Maintenance requirements of DCP per energy unit in the different Nordic countries.

Sweden	: 3 g DCP/0.5 MJ/$BW^{0.75}$	= 6 grams DCP/MJ
Denmark, Norway, Island	: 3 g DCP/0.0373 F.u/$BW^{0.75}$	= 80 grams DCP/F.u
Finland	: 3 g DCP/0.0429	= 70 grams DCP/ME (F.u)

4. Requirement for work

4.1 Energy

Energy requirement for work is difficult to describe in detail for different types of work. It is therefore proposed that the Nordic countries use the system described by NRC-89.

Energy requirement for work/training (percentage of maintenance requirement):
Light work : + 25%
Medium work : + 50%
Hard work : + 75%
Intense work : + 100%

4.2. Protein

Protein requirement for work is defined as DCP per energy unit. In Germany, France, USA and The Netherlands the DCP-content per unit energy for work is the same as for maintenance (Table 4).

Table 4. Requirement of DCP for work per energy unit in the different Nordic countries.

Sweden	: 3 g DCP/0.5 MJ/$BW^{0.75}$	= 6 grams DCP/MJ
Denmark, Norway, Island	: 3 g DCP/0.0373 F.u/$BW^{0.75}$	= 80 grams DCP/F.u
Finland	: 3 g DCP/0.0429	= 70 grams DCP/ME (F.u)

5. Requirement for pregnancy

Basis for the calculation of nutrient requirements for pregnancy is the definition of foetal growth. A foals body weight at birth is set to 10% of the BW of the mare. The growth of the foetus (% of birth weight) has been calculated in different ways. Table 5 gives the figures according to Meyer and Stadermann (1991).

Table 5. Growth and protein retention by the foetus.

Month of pregnancy	Growth of foetus (% of birth weight)	Protein retention (g/kg growth)
Total for month 1-7	19	101
8	10	148
9	18	192
10	23	168
11	30	213

In Holland these figures are being used when calculating the energy and protein requirements for pregnancy. The efficiency of protein conversion for pregnancy is set to 50%.

5.1 Energy

Energy requirement above maintenance is calculated for the 8., 9., 10., and 11. month of pregnancy. The basis for calculating the energy needs for pregnancy is the maintenance requirement, without any correction for breed. The percentage increase in energy requirement is somewhat higher for large horses than for the small breeds.

Table 6. Energy requirement for pregnancy, percentage of maintenance requirement.

	Month of pregnancy			
BW of mare	8	9	10	11
200 kg	5	11	15	21
500 kg	7	13	18	25
700 kg	7	14	20	28

It is suggested that the Nordic countries calculate the energy requirement for pregnancy according to the values for mares of 500 kg BW.

5.2 Protein

The protein requirement for pregnancy is a function of the growth of the foetus and the protein retention per kg growth.

Table 7. Protein requirement for pregnancy, (g/day).

Month of pregnancy	DCP- requirement	Example
8	12% of BW	DCP (g/d) for pregnancy for mare
9	25% of BW	500 kg in the 10. month of pregnancy:
10	33% of BW	DCP = 500 x 0.33 = 165 g/d
11	50% of BW	

Table 8. Calculation of protein requirement for pregnancy, g/day.

BW of mare	Month of pregnancy			
	8	9	10	11
200	24	50	66	100
300	36	75	105	150
400	48	100	132	200
500	60	125	165	250
600	72	150	198	300
700	84	175	231	350

6. Requirements for lactation

The requirement for lactation is calculated from the amount of milk produced and the composition of milk. Different values have been proposed for calculating a standard lactation curve for mares. According to the Dutch work, lactation is calculated according to table 9.

Table 9. Milk production during the lactation period in mares.

	Kg milk per 100 kg BW		
BW of mare	1. month of lact.	2-3 month of lact.	4-5 month of lact.
≤ 200	3.0	3.5	3.0
> 200	2.5	3.0	2.5

6.1 Energy

The energy requirement for milk production can be calculated from the energy content of milk and the amount of milk produced.

Table 10. Daily energy requirement for milk production per 100 kg BW.

Country	BW of mare, kg	Month of lactation		
		1	2 - 3	4 - 5
The Netherlands	≤ 200	960 VEP	970 VEP	790 VEP
	> 200	800 VEP	833 VEP	660 VEP
DK, N, Is	≤ 200	0.96 UFC	0.97 UFC	0.79 UFC
	> 200	0.80 UFC	0.83 UFC	0.66 UFC
Sweden	≤ 200	12.9 MJ	13.0 MJ	10.6 MJ
	> 200	10.8 MJ	11.2 MJ	8.9 MJ
Finland	≤ 200	1.10 F.u (ME)	1.11 F.u (ME)	0.91 F.u (ME)
	> 200	0.92 F.u (ME)	0.96 F.u (ME)	0.76 F.u (ME)

6.2 Protein

The protein requirement for milk production is calculated according to table 11.

Table 11. Calculation of protein requirement for lactation.

Month of lactation	Milk production, % of BW		Protein content g/kg milk	Efficiency of protein conversion	DCP g/kg milk
	BW ≤ 200	BW > 200			
1	3.0	2.5	25	50%	50
2	3.5	3.0	22	50%	44
3	3.5	3.0	22	50%	44
4	3.0	2.5	20	50%	40
5	3.0	2.5	20	50%	40

7. Requirements for growth

Requirement for growth is calculated from data on growth in young horses. In the Dutch work a standard growth curve for all types of horses is defined.

Table 12. Growth curve and body weight (kg) for young horses of different age and adult body weight.

Age (months)	0	3	6	9	12	15	18	21	14	27	30	33	36
% of BW_{adult}	10	30	47	58	67	75	82	86	89	92	94	96	97
BW_{adult}	Body weight of growing horse												
100	10	30	47	58	67	75	82	86	89	92	94	96	97
200	20	60	94	116	134	150	164	172	178	184	188	192	194
300	30	90	141	174	201	225	246	258	267	276	282	288	291
400	40	120	188	232	268	300	328	344	356	368	376	384	388
500	50	150	235	290	335	375	410	430	445	460	470	480	485
600	60	180	282	348	402	450	492	516	534	552	564	576	582
700	70	210	329	406	469	525	574	602	623	644	658	672	679
800	80	240	376	464	536	600	656	688	712	736	752	768	776

Table 13. Average daily gain (g/d) for young horses of different age and adult body weight.

Age (months)	3	6	9	12	15	18	21	24	27	30	33	36
% of BW_{adult}	30	47	58	67	75	82	86	89	92	94	96	97
BW_{adullt}	Weight gain (g/day)											
100	219	153	109	93	82	60	38	33	27	22	16	11
200	437	306	219	186	164	120	77	66	55	44	33	22
300	656	459	328	279	246	180	115	98	82	66	49	33
400	874	612	437	372	328	240	153	131	109	87	66	44
500	1093	765	546	464	410	301	191	164	137	109	82	55
600	1311	918	656	557	492	361	230	197	164	131	98	66
700	1530	1071	765	650	574	421	268	230	191	153	115	77
800	1749	1224	874	743	656	481	306	262	219	175	131	87

From the growth curve, average daily gain can be calculated dependent of age and adult body weight.

7.1 Energy

The energy requirement of young horses has two components, maintenance and growth. The maintenance requirement for young horses is higher than for fully grown horses.

Table 14. Maintenance energy requirement for young growing horses.

Age (months)	Energy requirement/ kg $BW^{0.75}$ /day		
	UFC	MJ (ME)	F.u (ME)
0 - 6	0.047	0.63	0.054
7 - 12	0.044	0.59	0.050
13 - 36	0.042	0.57	0.048

In the Dutch work, there is a detailed description of growth and the energy requirement for growth. For practical purposes a simple equation can be used to calculate the energy requirement for growth of young horses:

Table 15. Calculation of daily energy requirement for growth in young horses.

$Energy_{Growth}$ UFC	$= ADG \times (1350 + 67.94*Age - 1.093*Age^2)/1000$	(DK, N, Is)
$Energy_{Growth}$ MJ (ME)	$= ADG \times (1350 + 67.94*Age - 1.093*Age^2) \times 13.45 /1000$	(Sweden)
$Energy_{Growth}$ F.u (ME)	$= ADG \times (1350 + 67.94*Age - 1.093*Age^2) \times 13.45 /11700$	(Finland)

ADG = Average daily gain, kg
Age = Age in months

7.2 Protein

The protein requirement for growth is calculated from data on the rate of protein deposition at different age. The protein deposition per kg weight gain varies from about 200 g/kg at birth and declines to about 160 g/kg at 36 months of age.

The requirement for DCP can be calculated according to the equation:

$DCP_{Growth} = PD/0.45$ (in g/day)

PD = Protein deposition/day (Average daily gain x protein content (%) of gain).

On basis of the standard growth curve for young horses, total daily requirements for DCP can be calculated. Table 16 gives an example of the requirements for DCP, and the concentration of DCP/energy unit.

Table 16. Requirements for DCP (g/day), and the concentration of DCP/energy unit for young horses 6 months of age.

BW_{adult}	DCP	DCP/UFC	DCP/MJ(ME)	DCP/F.u(ME)
200	235	121	9.0	105
300	335	123	9.2	107
400	435	126	9.4	110
500	530	128	9.5	111
600	625	129	9.6	113
700	715	130	9.7	113

DCP/energy unit is higher for the larger breeds. This is because maintenance energy requirement is calculated from metabolic body weight.

For practical purposes the protein requirement/energy unit for horses with BW_{adult} = 500 kg can be used for all growing horses.

Table 17. Protein requirement (DCP, g/d) and DCP/energy unit for growing horses of different age.

Age, months	3	6	12	18	24	30	36
DCP, g/day	650	530	425	380	350	350	350
DCP/UFC	179	128	96	85	79	78	77
DCP/MJ(ME)	13.3	9.5	7.1	6.3	5.8	5.8	5.7
DCP/F.u(ME)	155	111	84	74	68	68	67

Lysine

The requirement for lysine for growing horses can be expressed as g/day, per kg dry matter, per 100g DCP or per energy unit. According to the Dutch work lysine requirement is 5.8, 5.0, and 4.5 g per 100 g DCP for foals 3, 6 and 12 months old, respectively. Table 18 gives lysine requirements calculated as g per energy unit.

Table 18. Lysine requirement (g/energy unit) for growing horses according to the Dutch recommendations.

Age, months	3	6	12
DCP/UFC, DK, N, Is	11	6	4.3
DCP/MJ (ME), Sweden	0.8	0.5	0.32
DCP/F.u (ME), Finland	9	6	4

These recommendations are a bit lower than the figures from NRC. For practical purposes it is suggested to use intermediate values in the Nordic countries (Table 19). These values are very close to the recommendations used at present.

Table 19. Lysine concentration (g/energy unit) for growing horses.

Age, months	3	6	12	18
DCP/f.u, DK, N, Is	11	7.5	5	5
DCP/MJ (ME), Sweden	0.8	0.6	0.45	0.45
DCP/F.u (ME), Finland	9	7	5	5

For young horses in training, the same lysine concentration is recommended per energy unit for work.

8. Feed evaluation

The energy content of feed is calculated according to the French equations. This gives the possibility to calculate energy as DE, ME and NE according to the standards in each country.

Protein content is calculated as DCP using digestibility values from experiments with horses or sheep.

A comparison of energy feeding systems for horses

Derek Cuddeford

University of Edinburgh, Scotland

1. Introduction

In a seminal review of the nutrition of the horse in 1955, Olsson and Ruudvere summarised the energy requirements of the horse for maintenance computed according to different authors and the systems available. At that time, systems were based on starch equivalent, Scandinavian feed units, feed units for ruminants, Russian oat feed units and total digestible nutrients (TDN). Since that time, the TDN system developed in the USA (Morrison, 1937) has given way to one based on digestible energy (NRC, 1989) which is used throughout North and South America, the UK, Australia, New Zealand, South East Asia and parts of Southern Europe. Over the last 18 years a new French Net Energy (NE) system has been developed and refined from that originally proposed (INRA, 1984). This system expresses the energy value of feeds in terms of horse feed units (Unite Fouragire Cheval; UFC); one feed unit is the net energy content (9.42 MJ) of one kg of barley used for maintenance. Another NE system, currently in use in the Netherlands, has feed values based on NE for milk production in ruminants (Smolders, 1990). The Scandinavian Feed Unit (ScFU) continues to be used in Denmark, whilst in Finland, Iceland and Norway, the Fattening Feed Unit (FFU) is in use. Both systems are based on digestibility trial values obtained with cattle and ruminant digestible crude protein (DCP) values are used as well. Protein-rich feeds have a higher energy value calculated in ScFU than in FFU (Staun, 1990). However, a feed or diet containing about 110 g of digestible protein per ScFU has the same calculated energy value in both units. The absence of data derived from experiments with horses in the Nordic countries precludes the use of a special feed unit for horses. Sweden is exceptional in that it has relied on a digestible energy (DE) system and is now using metabolisable energy (ME). In the USSR, the energy value of foodstuffs is based on the system derived by Kellner (1926) and expressed as Russian oat feed units; one unit (1 kg) corresponds to 0.6kg starch equivalent. The USSR also uses Energetic Feed Units (EFU) equivalent to 10.46 MJ ME (Memedeikin, 1990) which have been derived experimentally with horses. Spain, Portugal and Greece do not use any particular system, whereas Italy has moved from using the Leroy Fodder Unit to adopting the French UFC system in its entirety (Miraglia and Olivieri, 1990). More recently, it has been proposed (Austbø, 1996) that the Nordic countries adopt the French system as well. It is thus quite conceivable that in the near future, there will be only two systems of horse feeding practised and these will be based on DE according to the National Research Council (NRC, 1989) devised in the U.S.A. or NE (Vermorel and Martin-Rosset, 1997) as developed by INRA, France. In the meantime, the ScFU is still in use together with the Russian oat feed unit.

2. Feed energy values

2.1 DE-based

The NRC originally used TDN to describe the energy content of feed for horses. These units can be converted to DE since 1 kg TDN is equivalent to 4.4 Mcal DE (NRC, 1989) or 18.4 MJDE. This conversion factor was based on work with ruminants and the validity of its use has always been questionable. Particularly, in the light of results obtained in a small study with ponies by Barth *et al.* (1977) who estimated 19.246 MJ kg^{-1} for a hay or hay/concentrate diet; this value is 1.05 times greater than the proposed factor. Now, however, the current NRC tables use DE expressed as Mcal. The raison d'être for the NRC (1989) using DE is that little data exists for ME or NE values of horse feeds. Although it is preferable that DE values are determined by *in vivo* experimentation, equations are becoming available for the prediction of DE (see for example, Pagan, 1994). More recently, new technologies, such as *in vitro* gas production techniques have been developed and the data used to predict feed values ($r^2 = 0.72$; Lowman *et al.,* 1997). Whatever predictive methods are used, they require validation, a relatively simple procedure for DE but much more complicated for ME or NE.

2.1 NE-based

The NE system was introduced in France during 1984 by INRA because the DE system was considered to overvalue high-fibre feeds. The classic experiments of Wolff *et al.,* (1877a) showed that more digestible energy (15%) was required by the horse when fed a 75% hay diet compared to when fed a 75% cereal diet. Furthermore, (Vermorel and Martin-Rosset, 1997) showed that the DE requirements for maintenance and work were 25% higher when hay was fed compared to grain. Kronfeld (1996) developed a calorimetric model to derive heat production data for the utilisation of different diets by horses and showed clearly that fibre is thermogenic; replacement of fibre by cereal reduced the yield of heat. Thus, it follows that fibrous foods would be used less efficiently by the horse because of their greater heat increment. The NE system relies on maintenance being the major component of energy expenditure in horses (Martin-Rosset *et al.,* 1994) and that the NE value of nutrients depends on free energy being produced by oxidative processes (Vermorel *et al.,* 1984).

3. Energy requirements

For convenience, the American DE-based system will be referred to as NRC and the French NE-based system as INRA.

3.1 Maintenance

3.1.1 NRC

Derivation

The system devised in the United States was based on digestible energy (DE) and full details of it were published most recently in 1989 (NRC, 1989). Maintenance requirements were based on the work of Pagan and Hintz (1986a) who used four mature male animals weighing 125, 206, 500 and 856 kg to derive values. The previous publication by the National Research Council (NRC, 1978) used metabolic body size ($W^{0.75}$) in the calculation of maintenance energy requirements. This power function of liveweight was derived for interspecific comparisons (Brody, 1945; Schmidt-Nielson, 1984) and Kleiber (1961) proposed that the metabolic requirement of mammalian herbivores (MR in kcal day^{-1}) be related to liveweight as follows:

$$MR = 70\ W^{0.75} \quad (1)$$

where W is the weight of the animal in kg. However, intraspecific comparisons produce exponents for this relationship which are quite different from 0.75 (Thonney *et al.*, 1976). For example, Blaxter (1962) stated that the exponent was greater than 0.75 and as high as 0.90 when measuring metabolism of mature animals within a species. Pagan and Hintz (1986a) demonstrated that $W^{0.87}$ produced the best relationship between energy intake and energy balance. However, they also showed that the regression relationship between resting maintenance DE intake and body weight had a r^2 value of 0.999. Much earlier, Benedict (1938) had shown a linear relationship between fasting heat metabolism and liveweight. NRC (1989) uses the equation:

$$DE\ (Mcal\ day^{-1}) = 0.975 + 0.021\ W\ (W \text{ is weight in kg}) \quad (2)$$

that was derived by Pagan and Hintz (1986a) for stalled animals in a thermoneutral environment.

Activity allowance

Pagan and Hintz (1986a) cited the work of others (Breuer, 1968; Stillions and Nelson, 1972; Anderson *et al.*, 1983) and practical experience to justify the values for a 500 kg horse proposed by NRC (1978). This requirement was 29.1% higher than that predicted by equation (2) above, so Pagan and Hintz (1986a) arbitrarily increased the values predicted by this equation by multiplying them by a factor of 1.291 and so obtained a new equation:

$$DE\ (Mcal\ day^{-1}) = 1.375 + 0.03\ W \quad (3)$$

that was adjusted in NRC (1989) to:

$$DE\ (Mcal\ day^{-1}) = 1.4 + 0.03\ W \quad (4)$$

This equation allows for the energy required for 'normal' activity although the use of a single value across a range of liveweights is questionable. Equally, although no mass exponent is used and a linear relationship exists between energy requirements and liveweight, there is a large Y-intercept (1.4 Mcal) which will have an effect similar to that of a mass exponen

Heavy horses

It has been proposed (Potter *et al.*, 1987) that equation (4) overestimates the energy need of horses exceeding a mature weight of 600 kg. It is considered that they have a lower voluntary activity than lighter horses and are more docile. The equation for estimating maintenance requirements of horses weighing in excess of 600 kg is:

$$DE\ (Mcal\ day^{-1}) = 1.82 + 0.0383W - 0.000015W^2 \quad (5)$$

and the net result is that the energy requirements are reduced by 5, 10 and 15% at 700, 800 and 900 kg respectively compared to values obtained with equation (4). The somewhat arbitrary nature of these reductions is justified on the basis that the values obtained are consistent with other findings (NRC, 1989).

3.1.2 INRA

Derivation

Vermorel *et al.* (1984) reviewed the feeding trials that had been conducted with horses over the last century; see for example Wolff *et al.*, 1888; Breuer, 1968; Wooden *et al.*, 1970 and Stillions and Nelson, 1972. They concluded that the maintenance energy requirements amounted to 586 kJ DE, 502 kJ ME or 351 kJ NE $kg^{-1}\ W^{0.75}$. For a 500kg horse, NRC (1989) equation (2) gives a value of 48 MJ DE compared to a value of 62 derived using the French data. Table 1 illustrates the difference between the systems over a range of liveweights.

Table 1. Energy requirements (MJ d^{-1}) for maintenance of horses of varying liveweight using different energy systems and compared on a DE basis.

		liveweight (kg)		
		400	600	800
NRC (1989)	Equation (2)	39.2	56.8	74.4
	Equation (4)	56.1	81.2	106.3
	Equation (5)	-	-	95.8
Vermorel *et al.* (1984)		52.4	71.0	88.2

Activity allowance
Vermorel *et al.* (1984) suggest values whereby maintenance requirements should be increased depending on the type of horse and whether or not it has been working (see Table 2). It is generally accepted that the maintenance requirements of working animals are enhanced through an up-regulation of metabolic processes. Furthermore, temperament can effect requirements and this can be seen from Table 2 where Vermorel *et al.* (1984) indicate that bloodstock/Thoroughbreds have higher maintenance requirements.

Table 2. Factors for adjusting maintenance (m) requirements (factor x m): dependent on horse type and activity (After Vermorel et al., 1984).

Horse activity		Horse type		
		Draft	Riding	Bloodstock
At rest		1.00	1.05	1.10
In work		1.05	1.10	1.15
Stallion	– at rest	1.10	1.15	1.20
	– working	1.20-1.30	1.25-1.35	1.30-1.40

Application of the factor 1.10 to the maintenance needs of a 600 kg riding horse as shown in Table 2 raises the value from 71 (Table 1) to 78.1 MJ DE day^{-1} which is close to the NRC (1989) value of 81.2 MJDE.

3.2 Work

3.2.1 NRC

A mobile, open-circuit, indirect calorimetry system was used to determine the energy expended by four geldings weighing between 433 and 520 kg (Pagan and Hintz, 1986b). Energy expended was exponentially related to speed and proportional to the mass that was moved. DE requirements above maintenance are given by the following equation:

$$DE\ (kcal\ kg^{-1}\ h^{-1}) = \frac{[e^{(3.02+0.0065y)} - 13.92] \times 0.06}{0.57} \qquad (6)$$

where y is the speed m min^{-1}

However, requirements could only be reliably predicted for horses up to medium canter (350 m min^{-1}) and the equation would therefore only be appropriate for horses working aerobically for extended periods of time such as endurance horses. Earlier, Anderson *et al.* (1983) developed a quadratic equation to calculate the quantity of DE required for maintenance and work:

$$DE\ (Mcal\ d^{-1}) = 5.97 + 0.021W + 5.03X - 0.48X^2 \qquad (7)$$

($X = W$ (kg) x kilometres x 10^{-3})

The application of this equation is limited to situations where the workload (kg x kilometres) is less than 3560 which was the upper limit defined experimentally. Thus, the use of this equation is limited to those animals performing short periods of intense work such as sprint horses.

Analysis of feeding practices in racing yards etc indicates that horses consume up to 30 g dry feed kg^{-1} W (Glade, 1983) and, based on the feeds used, it has been estimated (NRC, 1989) that horses in intense work consume up to twice their maintenance DE requirement. Unlike ruminant production systems, output, in terms of work, is poorly defined and words such as "light", "medium" and "hard" abound when describing "work". There is little prospect of this unsatisfactory state of affairs being resolved since most horses in training are fed to maintain their weight and condition; the balance between forage and concentrate in the daily ration is adjusted according to "work" load which is judged in a fairly subjective fashion.

3.2.2 INRA

The energy costs of locomotion (kJ kg^{-1} h^{-1}) at different speeds have been calculated from those data published by a number of different authors, including Brody (1945), Thomas and Fregin (1981) and Hornicke *et al.* (1983). Their impact on DE requirements is shown in Table 3. There are no great differences between the NRC and French values although the latter serve to illustrate the variation between individuals in relation to their work energy requirement.

Table 3. The effect of speed of movement (m min-1) on DE requirement (kJ kg^{-1} h^{-1}) above maintenance.

"Work"	Speed	NRC (1978)	NRC (1989)	Vermorel *et al.*, (1984)
Walking	110	2.1	12.3	8.6-14.2
Slow trotting	200	21.3	27.0	20-40
Fast trotting	300	52.3	57.3	52-80
Cantering	350	100.0	87.8	59-92

Martin-Rosset *et al.*, (1994) considered that data obtained from feeding trials were more reliable than assessments based on oxygen consumption when estimating the energy costs of draught power. These authors relied on the data published by Olssen and Ruudvere (1955) who recalculated that obtained by Jespersen (1949) into Scandinavian Feed Units (ScFU); 0.5 and 1.0 units were required for one hour of medium and very heavy work respectively. One ScFU is equivalent to the net energy of 1kg of barley and thus is equivalent to 1 UFC. For an 800kg horse, NRC (1989) would increase the energy allowance by 9.58 MJ of DE, equating to about 0.74 UFC, for one hour of draught work.

4. Predicting feed values

4.1 In vivo

Metabolism studies are the classical means of determining apparently digestible nutrients; knowledge of endogenous losses enables the calculation of true digestibilities. Digestibility studies are easy to conduct and require minimal facilities. Collection of gas losses and urine from the animal enable the estimation of ME but this type of procedure requires calorimeters and so few estimations have been made with horses. One such study (Vermorel *et al.*, 1997) was used to provide supportive data for the French horse net energy system (Vermorel and Martin-Rosset, 1997) but relied on substantive assumptions in terms of the proportions of absorbed energy supplied by glucose and volatile fatty acids. Furthermore, it was assumed that DE and ME values of forages were similar when fed alone or in mixed diets. This assumption was based on the findings of Martin-Rosset and Dulphy (1987). Cuddeford *et al.*, (1992) showed a non-linear increase in ration energy digestibility as alfalfa was progressively substituted with naked oats. However, this could have been a "level of feeding effect" which might have affected the results of Vermorel *et al.*, (1997) because the rations they used were adjusted on an energy basis rather than by equalising DMI. Differences in the ME requirements for maintenance obtained in this study was explained on the basis of differences in the energy cost of eating, digestive tract metabolism and utilisation of digestion end products.

In vivo studies are the "gold standards" against which other methods of evaluating feeds are judged. Simultaneous *in vivo* digestibility trials in horses and wethers were used by Martin-Rosset *et al.,* (1984) to develop prediction equations so that *in vivo* ruminant data could be used to generate values for horses. The r^2 value for legumes was 0.71 with a residual standard deviation (RSD) of 2.6; comparable values for grasses were 0.96 and 2.3 respectively. Vander noot and Trout (1971) used *in vivo* studies in steers to predict values for horses and found that, not surprisingly, crude fibre was the best predictor of DMD ($r^2 = 0.81$). However, predictions based on *in vivo* studies in different species are prone to error and the INRA system is heavily dependent on such work.

4.2 Chemical composition of foods

Vermorel and Martin-Rosset (1997) were unable to reliably predict urine and methane losses and so predicted ME:DE ratios using two equations that relied on food composition:

$$\frac{ME\%}{DE} = 84.07 + 0.0165\ CF - 0.0276\ CP + 0.0184\ CC \qquad (8)$$

(CF = crude fibre; CP = crude protein; CC = cytoplasmic carbohydrates - all values in g kg^{-1} DM)

This equation underestimated ME:DE ratios of protein-rich feeds (>300 g CP kg^{-1}) so the following equation was used:

$$\frac{ME\%}{DE} = 94.36 - 0.011\ CF - 0.0275\ CP \qquad (9)$$

However, very low r^2 values, 0.45 and 0.17 respectively, were associated with these equations which must give cause for concern over their reliability. Martin-Rosset *et al.,* (1996a) used multiple regression to predict OMD of forages from their chemical composition and found that the following relationship could be used:

$$OMD(\%) = 67.78 + 0.07088\ CP - 0.000045\ NDF^2 - 0.12180\ ADL \qquad (10)$$

($r^2 = 0.878$)

These authors considered that this was a more reliable equation (RSD + 2.5) than that used earlier by Martin-Rosset *et al.,* (1984) which serves to illustrate the point that the INRA system can be improved.

5. Limitations

NRC (1989) maintenance energy requirements were calculated on the basis of experiments with four animals (Pagan and Hintz, 1986a) and from feeding trials which were the basis for NRC (1978). These feeding trials also provided the foundation for the INRA system (INRA, 1990) which has been subsequently validated (Vermorel *et al.,* 1997) using indirect calorimetry.

One UFC has a NE value of 9.414 MJ and is equivalent to 1 kg "standard barley" (sic) of 870 g DM kg^{-1} given to horses at maintenance. The justification for using maintenance as the basis for the feeding system is that it comprises the bulk of the energy need of different horses. For example, 0.50 to 0.90 of the total energy expended by lactating and pregnant mares respectively is for maintenance purposes (Doreau *et al.,* 1988), 0.60 to 0.90 in growing horses (Agabriel *et al.,* 1984) and 0.70 to 0.80 in working horses (Martin-Rosset *et al.,* 1994). However, in racehorses that are fed routinely at twice maintenance energy levels, the latter figures proposed for working horses are clearly wrong. The greatest differences in nutritive value between horse feeds are due to differences in OMD and are thus related to cell wall content or neutral detergent fibre (NDF). This is highly relevant since requirements are expressed in terms of DE or UFC; Table 4 illustrates the significance of this. It is clear that DE overvalues roughages however, large effects are only seen at the extremes of feed quality (c.f. maize with straw). Furthermore, since performance horses are fed diets containing a high proportion of concentrate (up to 0.70/0.80), the overvaluation of roughage DE is of little consequence. Vermorel and Martin-Rosset (1997) suggested that the NRC-DE system overvalued cereal by-products, oil meals and hays by about 0.15, 0.25-0.30 and 0.30-0.35 respectively; starch-rich feeds are undervalued. In practice, the bias introduced by a DE system is not great when mixed diets are fed.

It is assumed that the horse's need for different functions, such as work and maintenance, are additive. Thus, the daily energy need is arrived at using a factorial approach, summing the needs for both maintenance and work. The INRA system (INRA, 1990) assumes that the efficiency with which ME is used for different functions is the same as that for maintenance (km).

This means, for example, that the utilisation of ME for maintenance is the same as that for work (km = kw), however, the increased heat production associated with work may well invalidate this assumption. Using km to predict feed energy values for working animals will introduce errors. The relationships between the efficiency of utilisation of ME for maintenance and pregnancy and lactation may be similar as in ruminants but, apart from draught work, there is no analogous basis for a relationship between maintenance and work in ruminants as in horses. Indeed, it is unlikely that nutrient utilisation for work will be particularly efficient.

The INRA system (INRA, 1990) assumes that the NE requirements of horses in different situations have been accurately described but this is not the case. Validation experiments have only been conducted at or near maintenance (Vermorel and Vernet, 1991; Vermorel *et al.,* 1997).

The INRA system assumes that UFC's are additive (Martin-Rosset and Dulphy, 1987) based on digestibility data. However, the system relies on estimating absorbed energy by predicting which nutrients are absorbed. No account is taken of feed interactions or, in other words, how different feeds and the way in which they are fed, affects the site of digestion, extent of digestion and the resultant nutrient uptake. It has been demonstrated (Potter *et al.,* 1992; Meyer *et al.,* 1993) that both the dietary origin of starch and the manner in which it has been processed are important. These

Table 4. DE (MJ kg^{-1} DM) and UFC (kg^{-1} DM) values of some common feeds and, as a proportion of maize.

Feed	DE	DE feed DE maize	UFC	UFC feed UFC maize
Maize	16.1	1.00	1.33	1.00
Barley	14.5	0.90	1.16	0.87
Oats	12.5	0.78	0.99	0.74
Beet pulp	12.5	0.78	0.86	0.65
Lucerne	10.2	0.63	0.60	0.45
Grass hay	7.4	0.46	0.44	0.33
Barley straw	6.5	0.40	0.36	0.27

factors will affect both the site of digestion and the magnitude of pre-caecal digestion and the latter will have a major impact on whether glucose or VFA is the substrate for subsequent ATP production. Recent work (McLean *et al.,* unpublished) has shown that processing barley by micronising or extrusion affects pre-caecal starch degradation, the molar proportions of VFA in the caecum as well as the caecal pH; all factors that could affect km values. Moore-Colyer *et al.,* (1997a, b) have shown that considerable quantities of non-starch polysaccharide (up to 149 g kg^{-1}) can disappear pre-caecally and as a consequence, this will affect the proportion of nutrients absorbed from the lumen of the hindgut. Thus, until such time as those factors (for example size of meal, rate of passage of feed residues, etc) that affect the magnitude and site of nutrient uptake have been defined, the putative assumptions should be interpreted with care. In contrast, Vermorel and Martin-Rosset (1997) assert that large errors in the estimation of nutrient uptake have small effects on km (0.004) although how efficiency is affected in terms of productive function is not disclosed.

The NE of barley is deduced from the assumption that it contains 16.13 MJ GE kg^{-1} and has a DM of 870 g kg^{-1}. The NE is determined by a step-wise procedure assuming the following relationships: DE/GE = 0.80, ME/DE = 0.931 and NE/ME = 0.785. The validity of using these conversion factors has been questioned (Harris, 1997) particularly as the NE value is assumed to be constant for whatever purpose the food energy is being used. The function of the animal, environment, nutrient content of the ration and other factors will affect the NE value of a food. For practical rations composed of 0.75 forage and 0.25 concentrate, Tisserand (1988) suggests the following relationships between energy values: DE/GE = 0.67-0.83, ME/DE = 0.83-0.91 and NE/ME = 0.63-0.80. With this magnitude of variation, it is difficult to accept that UFC values are additive (Martin-Rosset and Dulphy, 1987). Indeed, it seems to be a retrograde step to use a feed unit that has no dimension, in place of absolute energy values; the justification given is that feeds are more frequently compared in terms of substitution value.

In summary, a DE system relies on digestibility as the most important factor for discriminating between feeds. An NE system separates concentrates and roughages and is based on end-product usage. As well as considering the efficiency of utilisation of these end-products (glucose, lactate, VFA etc.), an NE system quantifies the impact of the energy costs of mastication, propulsion of food through the gut and heat of fermentation on km. For example, the km for barley might be 0.79 compared to only 0.60 for grass hay. Ultimately, however, the practical value of a feeding system will depend upon the reliability of feed evaluation methodologies and in this context, roughages, succulents and fresh forages are poorly defined.

It is perhaps salutary to record the comments of Hintz and Cymbaluk (1994) who noted that direct comparisons between the NRC and INRA systems cannot be made easily or without several assumptions. Furthermore, the calculations, based on either system, when expressed in feed rather than in terms of DE, UFC's etc. produced similar values. They took the example of a lactating, 500kg mare and, in spite of using different energy units, the final rations were similar. Frape (1998) compared the two systems for ration formulation and concluded that:

1. expected selection against poor hay by the NE system did not occur;
2. the DE system generally assumed higher requirements for different functions, which offset the higher values given to hay;
3. a change in assumed feed intake of working horses had a large effect on ration composition with either system.

The INRA system is flexible and can be modified and up-dated as new information comes to hand although at present, it's complexity compared to NRC, does not appear to confer any major advantage. Furthermore, the extent of its assumptions and the lack of experimental data do not support the widespread adoption of an NE system for rationing performance horses.

References

Agabriel, J., Martin-Rosset, W. and Robelin, J., 1984. Croissance et besoins du poulain. In: R. Jarrige and W. Martin-Rosset (Editors), Le Cheval, Reproduction, Sélection, Alimentation, Exploitation. INRA Publications, Route de St Cyr, 78000 Versailles, pp. 371-384.

Anderson, C.E., Potter, G.D., Kreider, J.L. and Courtney, C.C., 1983. Digestible energy requirements for exercising horses. Journal of Animal Science, 56: 91-95.

Austbø, D., 1996. Energy and protein evaluation systems and nutrient recommendations for horses in the Nordic countries. In: Proceedings of the 47th E.A.A.P. Meeting. Lillehammer, Norway, p. 293

Barth, K.M., Williams, J.W. and Brown, D.G., 1977. Digestible energy requirements of working and non-working ponies. Journal of Animal Science, 44: 585-589.

Benedict, F.G., 1938. Vital Energetics. Carnegie Institute, Washington DC, Pub. No. 503.

Blaxter, K.L., 1962. The Energy Metabolism of Ruminants. Hutchison & Co. Ltd., London.

Breuer, L.H., 1968. Energy nutrition of the light horse. In: Proceedings of the 1st Equine Nutrition and Physiology Symposium. University of Kentucky, Lexington, p. 8.

Brody, S., 1945. Bioenergetics and growth. Hafner Pub. Co. New York.

Cuddeford, D., Khan, N. and Muirhead, R., 1992. Naked oats - an alternative energy source for performance horses. In: Proceedings of the 4th International Oat Conference. Adelaide, South Australia, pp. 42-50.

Doreau, M., Martin-Rosset, W. and Boulot, S., 1988. Energy requirements and the feeding of mares during lactation: A review. Livestock Production Science, 20: 53-68.

Frape, D., 1998. Equine Nutrition and Feeding, 2nd ed. Blackwell Science Ltd., London.

Glade, M.J., 1983. Nutrition and performance of racing thoroughbreds. Equine Veterinary Journal, 15: 31-36.

Harris, P., 1997. Energy sources and requirements of the exercising horse. Annual Review of Nutrition, 17: 185-210.

Hintz, H.F. and Cymbaluk, N.F., 1994. Nutrition of the horse. Annual Review of Nutrition, 14: 243-267.

Hörnicke, H., Meixner, R. and Pollmann, R., 1983. Respiration in exercising horses. In: Equine exercise physiology, (eds) D.H. Snow, S.G.B. Persson and R.J. Rose, Granta Edition. Cambridge, pp. 7-16.

INRA, 1984a. Tables des apports alimentaires recommandés pour le cheval. In: R. Jarrige, W. Martin-Rosset (eds). Le Cheval, Reproduction, Sélection, Alimentation, Exploitation. INRA Publications, Route de St Cyr, 78000 Versailles, pp. 645-660.

INRA, 1990. L'alimentation des chevaux. W. Martin-Rosset (ed). INRA Publications, Route de St Cyr, 78000 Versailles.

Jespersen, J., 1949. Normes pour les besoins des animaux: chevaux, porcs et poules. In: Vème Congrès International de Zootechnie, Paris, Vol 2, Rapports Particuliers, pp. 33-43.

Kellner, O., 1926. The Scientific Feeding of Farm Animals, 2nd edn (translated by W. Goodwin), London, Duckworth.

Kleiber, M., 1961. The Fire of Life. John Wiley and Sons, Inc., New York, NY.

Lowman, R.S., Theodorou, M.K., Dhanoa, M.S., Hyslop, J.J. and Cuddeford, D., 1977. Evalution of an in vitro gas production technique for estimating the in vivo digestibility of equine feeds. In: Proceedings of the 15th Equine Nutrition and Physiology Symposium, Forth Worth, Texas, pp. 1-2.

Martin-Rosset, W. and Dulphy, J.P., 1987. Digestibility interactions between forages and concentrates in horses: influence of feeding level-comparison with sheep. Livestock Production Science, 17: 263-276.

Martin-Rosset, W., Andrieu, J. and Jestin, M., 1996a. Prediction of the organic matter digestibility (OMD) of forages in horses from the chemical composition. In: Proceedings of the 47th E.A.A.P. Meeting, Lillehammer, Norway. p. 295 (abs).

Martin-Rosset, W., Andrieu, J., Vermorel, M. and Dulphy, J.P., 1984. Valeur nutritive des aliments pour le cheval. In: R. Jarrige and W. Martin-Rosset (Editors), Le Cheval, Reproduction, Sélection, Alimentation, Exploitation. INRA Publications, Route de St Cyr, 78000 Versailles, pp 208-238.

Martin-Rosset, W., Vermorel, N., Doreau, M., Tisserand, J.L. and Andrieu, J., 1994. The French horse feed evaluation systems and recommended allowances for energy and protein. Livestock Production Science, 40: 37-56.

Memedeikin, V.G., 1990. The energy and nitrogen systems used in the USSR for horses. In: Proceedings of the 41st E.A.A.P. Meeting, Toulouse, France. p 382 (abs).
Miraglia, N. and Olivieri, O., 1990. Statement and expression of the energy and nitrogen value of feedstuffs in Southern Europe. In: Proceedings of the 41st E.A.A.P. Meeting, Toulouse, France. p. 390 (abs).
Moore-Colyer, M.J.S., Hyslop, J.J., Longland, A.C. and Cuddeford, D., 1997a. Degradation of four dietary fibre sources by ponies as measured by the mobile bag technique. In: Proceedings of the 15th Equine Nutrition and Physiology Symposium, Fort Worth, Texas. pp. 118-119.
Moore-Colyer, M.J.S., Hyslop, J.J., Longland, A.C. and Cuddeford, D., 1997b. The degradation of organic matter and crude protein of four botanically diverse feedstuffs in the foregut of ponies as measured by the mobile bag technique. In: Proceedings of the British Society of Animal Science. p. 120.
Morrison, F.B., 1937. Feeds and Feeding. Handbook for the Student and Stockman, 20th edition. Ithaca, N.Y.
NRC, 1978. Nutrient Requirements of Horses, (4th Revised Edition). National Academy of Sciences, Washington DC.
NRC, 1989. Nutrient Requirements of Horses, (5th Revised Edition). National Academy of Sciences, Washington DC.
Olsson, N.A. and Ruudvere, A., 1955. The nutrition of the horse. Nutrition Abstracts and Reviews, 25: 1-18.
Pagan, J.D., 1994. Digestibility trials provide evaluation of feedstuffs. Feedstuffs 66: 14-15.
Pagan, J.D. and Hintz, H.F., 1986a. Equine energetics. 1. Relationship between bodyweight and energy requirements in horses. Journal of Animal Science, 63: 815-821.
Pagan, J.D. and Hintz, H.F., 1986b. Equine energetics. II. Energy expenditure in horses during submaximal exercise. Journal of Animal Science, 63: 822-830.
Potter, G.D., Gibbs, P.G., Haley, R.G. and Klenshoj, C., 1992. Digestion of protein in the small and large intestine of equines fed mixed diets. In: Pferdeheilkunde, September 1992, ISSN 0177-7726. pp. 140-143.
Schmidt-Nielsen, K., 984. Scaling: Why animal size is so important. Cambridge University Press, Cambridge.
Smolders, E.A.A., 1990. Evolution of the energy and nitrogen systems used in The Netherlands. In: Proceedings of the 41st E.A.A.P. Meeting, Toulouse, France. p. 386 (abs).
Staun, H., 1990. Energy and nitrogen systems used in northern countries for estimating and expressing value of feedstuffs in horses. In: Proceedings of the 41st E.A.A.P. Meeting, Toulouse, France. p. 388 (abs).
Stillions, M.C. and Nelson, W.E., 1972. Digestible energy during maintenance of the light horse. Journal of Animal Science, 34: 981-982.
Thomas, D.P. and Fregin, G.F., 1981. Cardiorespiratory and metabolic response to treadmill exercise in the horse. Pfl(gers Archives, 385: 65-70.
Thonney, M.L., Touchberry, R.W., Goodrich, R.D. and Meiske, J.C., 1976. Intraspecies relationship between fasting heat production and body weight: A re-evaluation of $W^{.75}$. Journal of Animal Science, 43: 692-704.
Tisserand, J.L., 1988. Nutrition of the Non-Ruminant Herbivores - Horses. Livestock Production Science, 19: 279-288.
Vander noot, G.W. and Trout, J.R., 1971. Prediction of digestible components of forages by equines. Journal of Animal Science, 33: 38-41.
Vermorel, M. and Martin-Rosset, W., 1997. Concepts, scientific bases structures and validation of the French horse net energy system (UFC). Livestock Production Science, 47: 261-275.
Vermorel, M. and Vernet, J., 1991. Energy utilisation of digestion end-products for maintenance in ponies. In: Energy metabolism of farm animals, eds. C. Wenk and M. Boessinger. E.A.A.P. Publication Number 58. pp 433-436.
Vermorel, M., Jarrige, R. and Martin-Rosset, W., 1984. Métabolisme et besoins énergétiques du cheval, le système des UFC. In: R. Jarrige and W. Martin-Rosset (Editors), Le Cheval, Reproduction, Sélection, Alimentation, Exploitation. INRA Publications, Route de St Cyr, 87000 Versailles. pp. 239-276.
Wolff, E., Funke, W., Kreuzhage, C. and Kellner, O., 1877a. Pferde Futterungsversuche. Landwirtsch, Versuch, Stu., 20: 125-168.
Wooden, G.R., Knox, K.L. and Wild, C.L., 1970. Energy metabolism of light horses. Journal of Animal Science, 30: 544-548.

Voluntary food intake by horses

Derek Cuddeford

University of Edinburgh, Scotland

1. Controls

It is not known whether the controls of intake are the same for horses and ponies, different sexes or for different breed types. Given the opportunity, non-working horses and ponies will eat in excess of their energy needs and, as a result, become obese. Ralston (1992) reported an attempt to stabilise intake and body weight in horse mares fed a pelleted diet *ad libitum*. However, animals continued to gain weight and consume all feed offered over a five-week period so the experiment was terminated on the grounds that the animals were becoming obese. There appears to be some sensitivity to energy intake in that ponies ate larger meals more frequently when offered a pelleted diet of a reduced energy density (Laut, Houpt, Hintz and Houpt, 1985) than when they were fed a standard pelleted diet. The ponies' response to changes in dietary energy density took between two and 14 days to stabilise indicating a less precise mechanism than that present in other species (rats and monkeys) where compensation occurs in less than 24 h (Gibbs and Smith, 1978). However, ponies were able to compensate intake of the pelleted diet that they were accustomed to when given additional intragastric inputs of energy in the form of glucose, corn oil or α-cellulose accurately, within a 24 h period (Ralston and Baile, 1982b; 1983).

Some feedback mechanisms appear to affect food intake by ponies. Ralston and Baile (1983) showed that reductions in intake occurred at times that would reflect the post-absorptive state; 10 to 15 minutes for glucose and 4 to 6h for cellulose. An intra-gastric load of corn oil immediately after a 4h fast, and before a meal, did not affect consumption of the meal but did reduce subsequent intake by tripling the normal inter-meal interval. This could have resulted from metabolic feedback or a reduced rate of gastric emptying. Ralston and Baile (1982a) concluded that elevated levels of plasma glucose and insulin do not immediately generate satiety cues in ponies, although this view was based on glucose infusions via the jugular vein. Such an infusion would enable utilisation of the metabolite and possibly, reduce effects at receptor sites. It is noteworthy that the glucose would probably have by-passed liver receptors as well.

The effect of gut fill on intake is equivocal. Intra-gastric infusions of kaolin had no significant effect on DMI or feeding behaviour of ponies when compared with control animals (Ralston and Baile, 1982b). These authors suggested that stomach fill had no effect on intake although this ignores the fact that kaolin is inert and that it would not generate stimuli analogous to those produced by feed residues. Removal of 1.2 to 1.5 l of caecal contents (equivalent to 0.22 of total caecal content of a 200kg pony) also had no effect on subsequent feeding behaviour of ponies (Ralston, Freeman and Baile, 1983). However, intra-gastric infusions of α-cellulose significantly ($p<0.05$) reduced total DMI after 3 to 18 h post-infusion (Ralston and Baile, 1982b). Both of these results need to be interpreted with care because removal of a small amount of digesta is unlikely to have had much effect on intake and in the case of α-cellulose, it could have had a "fill" effect, a metabolite effect or both. In fact, Ralston and Baile (1982a) suggested that intra-gastric loads of nutrients generate satiety cues in ponies that are not related to the volume or bulk of the treatment. For example, a control infusion of 2 l of water had no effect on feeding behaviour whereas 2 l of water containing 300g of dissolved glucose decreased intakes 0 to 3 h post-treatment. This probably represents a post-absorptive effect rather than a localised gastric response because of its duration. However, the tonicity of the solution would have affected fluid balance that in itself, could have had an effect. NDF apparent digestibility and NDF content of feed are not reliable predictors of DMI ($r^2 = 0.266$) in horses (Cymbaluk, 1990) suggesting that physical capacity of the large intestine is unlikely to limit feed intake. However, if faecal output is a determinant of DMI then large intestinal capacity may have a role in controlling intake. The flow of digesta through the horse's GIT is slowed but it is not limited by particle size in the same way as it is in ruminants since there is no analogous structure to the reticulo-omasal orifice. Thus, digesta cannot be retained in the horse's GIT in the same way that it can in ruminants and therefore, there is less likelihood of "fill" negatively affecting intake.

Intra-gastric infusion of acetate (0.75mmol/kg W) caused ponies to increase feed intake ($p<0.05$) by reducing the duration of the first inter-meal interval (Ralston *et al.*, 1983). Intravenous studies with short chain, volatile fatty acids have not been undertaken and as a result, it is not known how circulating levels of these acids may affect voluntary feed intake. Following a 4 h fast, above normal levels of acetate (1.0 and 1.25mmol/kg W) and propionate (0.75mmol/kg W) were introduced as a bolus into the caecum of ponies and reduced feed intake, manifest by prolonging the first inter-meal interval (Ralston *et al.*, 1983). An intra-caecal infusion of 0.4mol propionate/kg W significantly ($p<0.05$) increased total feed intake by 1.075 relative to control values. In contrast, an infusion of 1mmol propionate/kg W significantly ($p<0.01$) reduced by 0.22, the size of the first meal consumed without affecting subsequent feeding behaviours. However, the relevance of this type of research, that relied on the provision of complete pelleted diets fed *ad libitum* and consumed in 10/11 meals/24h, to the intake of an *ad libitum* forage-fed horse or pony is questionable.

In summary, there is a dearth of facts relating to intake controls in horses although Ralston (1984) concluded that horses rely primarily on oro-pharyngeal and external stimuli to control the size and duration of an isolated meal. She considered that meal frequency is regulated by the presence and/or absorption of the products of digestion together with metabolic cues that may reflect body energy stores. However, the influence of the latter may be deemed weak in view of the fact that fat ponies tend to get fatter!

2. Estimates of feed intake

Various attempts have made to measure the voluntary intake of different feeds by horses and ponies and to derive means whereby intake may be predicted. The foregoing represents a summary of this work and serves to illustrate how the equid responds to the different forms and characteristics of feed in a way that is quite different from that of ruminants.

2.1 Hay

The voluntary DMI's of a wide variety of hays have been measured and attempts made to establish the relationship between hay type, fibre content (defined as NDF and ADF) and voluntary DMI (see Table 1). Aiken, Potter, Conrad and Evans (1989), fed Coastal Bermuda grass to both yearlings and mature geldings, and suggested that food intake was regulated by energy requirement, rather than by gut capacity. This was based on the fact that the yearlings, with higher nutrient need, consumed more DM *pro rata* than the mature horses; 0.025 versus 0.02 of body weight. This is in keeping with the view proposed by Frape, Tuck, Sutcliffe and Jones (1982), based on a comparitive study with a pony, horse and white rhino, that voluntary DMI was proportionate to energy requirement rather than gut volume.

Comparisons of the voluntary DMI of chopped hays (legume and grass) by Arabian geldings (Crozier, Allen, Jack, Fontenot and Cochran, 1997) led to the conclusion that the higher intakes

Table 1. Relationship between hay type, fibre content and voluntary dry matter intake.

Hay Type	Age of horse	Content (g/kg DM)		Voluntary dry matter intake (g/kg W $^{0.75}$)	Apparent digestibility coefficient		Reference
		NDF	ADF		NDF	ADF	
Coastal bermuda	Yearlings	704.5	319.0	111.5	0.45	0.40	Aitken et al., (1989)
	Mature geldings			95.6	0.46	0.36	
Alfalfa	Arabian geldings	550	430	122	0.47	0.45	Crozier et al., (1997)
Tall fescue		720	400	111	0.44	0.37	
Caucasian bluestem		730	390	102	0.41	0.33	
Altai wildrye	Horses	749	-	81.2	-	-	Cymbaluk (1990)
Bromegrass		595	-	113.6	-	-	
Crested wheatgrass		689	-	85.0	-	-	
Kentucky bluegrass		727	-	82.3	-	-	
Oat hay		685	-	81.2	-	-	
Reed canary grass		655	-	99.4	-	-	
Long alfalfa hay		614	-	114.4	-	-	
Dehydrated alfalfa pellets		439	-	97.9	-	-	
Mature, threshed grass hay	Ponies	796	488	95.6	0.28	0.30	Hyslop et al., (1998)
High temperature dehydrated grass	Mature ponies	677	300	110	0.51	0.34	Hyslop et al., (1998)
Hay		695	332	113	0.40	0.26	
Alfalfa	Mature horse geldings	535		111			Dulphy et al., (1997a)
		563		92			
Regrowth grass		641		110			
		672		95			
Early cut grass hay		665		115			
		628		104			
Normal cut grass hay		663		111			
		655		99			
Late cut grass hay		702		102			
		709		100			

($p<0.05$) of legume hay, compared to grass hays were a reflection of its significantly higher ($p<0.01$) dry matter digestibility.

Cymbaluk (1990) compared a number of Canadian grass hays, fed *ad libitum* to horses, with long alfalfa hay and dehydrated alfalfa pellets. It appeared that horses voluntarily consumed more alfalfa hay than grass hay although there was no explanation for this phenomenon. Ponies offered *ad libitum* mature, threshed grass hay by Hyslop, Tomlinson, Bayley and Cuddeford (1998) were able to consume relatively large amounts of dry matter, even though this hay was of very poor quality (dry matter digestibility [DMD], 0.30). These results support the view that there is a poor relationship between intake and the cell wall content of hays. A further experiment (Hyslop, Bayley, Tomlinson and Cuddeford, 1998) examined the effect of the method of conservation on the voluntary feed intake of grass products by mature ponies. Although the hay was of poorer quality, more was consumed; the difference in intake was non-significant but the difference in NDF digestibility was ($p<0.01$). A comparative study in France (Dulphy, Martin-Rosset, Dubroeucq, Ballet, Detour and Jailler, 1997a) with mature horse geldings showed very similar voluntary DMI's for different hays. Alfalfa, re-growth grass, early cut, normal cut and late cut grass hays were fed in two trials. The authors concluded that because the horses consumed the different hays in practically the same amounts, it would be difficult to define precise criteria whereby it would be possible to predict likely intakes of dry forages by horses. A retrospective analysis of data obtained by INRA (Theix) and of values taken from published papers provided a data set for assessing voluntary DMI of horses fed different dry forages (Dulphy, Martin-Rosset, Dubroeucq and Jailler, 1997b). The pooled results for horses gave DMI's for legumes (n=12), grasses (n=38) and re-growth grass hays (n=7) of 108, 93 and 98g/kg$W^{0.75}$ respectively; the only significant ($p<0.05$) difference was between legume and grass hay. The authors concluded that voluntary intake of horses was not influenced by either the CP, crude fibre (CF) or NDF content of the forage. Multiple regression analysis yielded r^2 values between 0.11 and 0.13; in contrast, r^2 values for sheep calculated under similar conditions produced significant correlations of 0.78 to 0.84. Thus, it is impossible to reliably predict the intake of dry hays by horses based on forage analysis in contrast to ruminants, where effective equations have been derived and are based primarily on fibre content. Thus, Dulphy *et al.*, (1997b) have proposed that the voluntary intake of hays by housed, mature light horses will be in the range 19-22, 18-21 and 22-25g/kgW for grass, re-growth grass and alfalfa hays respectively. These values may be regarded as conservative estimates of voluntary DMI by horses. It seems to be a consistent finding that the intakes of legume hays are higher than that of grass hays and this may be for the reasons proposed by Minson (1990) to account for the higher intake of legumes by ruminants. He proposed that legumes had lower values for resistance to physical breakdown, percentage of cell wall, length-to-width ratios of fibres and energy required for mastication compared to grasses. It is noteworthy that the inclusion of soaked unmolassed sugar beet pulp in a daily ration can significantly ($p<0.05$) depress the voluntary intake of hay by ponies so that the maximum recommended inclusion of dry product is 0.3kg/day/100kgW (Hyslop and Cuddeford, 1999). The nature of this interaction is not known.

A recent review (Lawrence, Lawrence and Coleman, 2001) of published studies that reported both NDF and voluntary DMI (VDMI) in mature horses fed long stem grass hays *ad libitum* concluded that there was a good relationship between the two parameters represented by:

$$\text{VDMI (y)}=124.55+0.0155x^2-2.5742x \ (r^2=0.67,\ p<0.001) \quad (1)$$
(x=%NDF; y=g/kgW/day)

These authors tested the reliability of this equation in terms of predicting intake by feeding two orchard grass and two timothy hays to 4 mature equids (278-705kg). Predicted daily intakes were not significantly different from actual intakes and in fact, the two were highly correlated ($r^2=0.86$, $p<0.001$). Incorporation of the experimental data into that derived from the literature (1) yielded:

$$\text{VDMI (y)}=80.954+0.0073x^2-1.3677x \ (r^2=0.50,\ p<0.01;\ n=21) \quad (2)$$

It is apparent from these data that, whilst NDF may have a role in determining *ad libitum* intake of hays, there are clearly other factors involved.

2.2 Fresh herbage

There is a paucity of information in relation to the voluntary intake of fresh forage by horses, but that which is available is detailed in Table 2.

Dulphy *et al.*, (1997b) in their review, included data for 16 fresh forages (covering a range of NDF from 300 to 611g/kgDM) and obtained a mean intake figure similar to that for grass hays whose NDF content varied from 495 to 709g/kgDM. Published values for fresh forages (examined by Dulphy *et al.*, 1997b) varied between 90 and 117, with a mean of 105gDM/kgW$^{.75}$, not that dissimilar from the data derived from the INRA studies. As a result of these analyses, these authors suggested a probable fresh forage (grass) voluntary intake of 19-22gDM/kgW.

An interesting aspect of recent work in New Zealand (Grace, Gee, Firth and Shaw, 2002; Grace, unpublished), was that when pasture was cut and fed to horses in order to measure apparent DM digestibility *in vivo*, DMI was lower than when grazing. The depression was 0.10-0.15 in stalled yearlings and 0.05-0.08 in corralled mares; both groups were offered about 0.30 excess herbage. This work investigated the pasture intakes of yearlings and lactating brood mares and was based on faecal collection off the pasture and an *in vivo* assessment of pasture digestibility. This outcome illustrated the importance of grazing preference and its effect on voluntary DMI. Pasture intake data obtained in Australia (McMeniman, 2000) using alkane markers and Australian Stockhorse weanlings, produced similar results to those obtained in New Zealand. Further Australian work with thoroughbred weanlings (Friend and Nash, 2000) used similar markers but obtained unreliable estimates of intake (100gOM/kgW). These overestimates were thought to be as a result of pasture sampling errors but were probably also a result of too infrequent dosing of alkane. These types of problem further highlight the difficulty of conducting pasture intake studies.

Table 2. Estimates of voluntary dry matter intake of pasture by horses.

Pasture	Horse type	NDF Content (g/kgDM)	Voluntary dry matter intake	Reference
Fresh forage	Horses	300 - 611	97 g/kg W $^{0.75}$	Dulphy *et al.* (1997b)
Fresh forages		-	105 g/kg W $^{0.75}$	Dulphy *et al.* (1997b)
Fresh grass (Predicted)		-	19 - 22 g DM/kgW	
Pasture, grazed	Yearlings	-	85g/kg W $^{0.75}$	Grace et al. (2001)
	Lactating, brood mares	-	118 g/kg W $^{0.75}$	
Pasture	Australian stockhorse weanlings	-	20 - 30 gDM/kgW	McMeniman (2000)
Pasture	Thoroughbred weanlings	-	100g OM/kgW	Friend and Nash (2000)

2.3 Straws

The relationship between straw type, fibre content and VDMI of horses has been estimated by a number of workers, and comparisons drawn between the VDMI of straws and other forages (see Table 3).

Table 3. Relationship between straw type, fibre content and voluntary dry matter intake of horses.

Straw type	Horse type	NDF Content	Voluntary dry matter intake	Reference
Barley straw	Mature gelded horses	817 - 830	43 -46 gDM/kg W $^{0.75}$	Dulphy *et al.*, (1997a)
Straws	-	-	61 gDM/kg W $^{0.75}$	Dulphy *et al.*, (1997b)
Straw	Adult, light horses at maintenance		11 - 14 gDM/kgW	Dulphy *et al.*, (1997b)
Alfalfa Alfalfa/Oat Straw Alfalfa/Oil/Yeast			79.5 gDM/kg W $^{0.75}$ 73.3 gDM/kg W $^{0.75}$ 77.7 gDM/kg W $^{0.75}$	Hyslop and Calder, 2001

Dulphy *et al.*, (1997a) measured the voluntary DMI of barley straw by mature, gelded horses to be approximately half that of grass hays. Pearson and Merritt (1991) had previously reported a similar situation in resting donkeys; 80.9 and 36.8gDM/kgW$^{.75}$/day respectively for hay and barley straw. However, the difference was not so great in resting ponies, 99.1 and 59.8 and surprisingly, the ponies appeared to be better able to compensate the poor quality forage offered. Pearson, Archibald and Muirhead (2001) reported that the voluntary DMI of oat straw by ponies was reduced by about 0.40 compared to when the ponies were fed *ad libitum* artificially dehydrated alfalfa. Similarly, Dulphy *et al.*, (1997b) reported a pooled intake value for undefined straws by adult light horses at maintenance that was rather lower than that reported for other dry forages. Thus, horses do not appear to be able to effectively compensate lower feed energy densities by eating more, although there is no evidence to support the view that intake is limited by the capacity of the GIT. Longer MRT's may inhibit intake although they may in themselves be a result of low intakes furthermore, rate of elimination from the hindgut may have an impact on intake. Low intake of "cereal straw" must be influenced by its low palatability, a complex of organoleptic qualities including taste, structure, texture and smell. However, results recently reported by Hyslop and Calder (2001) showed that the inclusion of approximately 0.50 oat straw in a short-chopped, dehydrated and molassed alfalfa diet had very little effect on total DMI. Thus, it would seem that the voluntary intake of straw by horses can be markedly affected by the inclusion of other dietary ingredients (perhaps supplying fermentable energy and nitrogen) and that perhaps, the type of straw also has an impact on intake. An alternative explanation for low intakes of straw could be that the rate of comminution falls as the quality of the diet declines (Forbes, 1988) so a poorer quality diet, such as straw, takes longer to eat. In addition, longer inter-meal intervals are required and if time spent feeding is an important feedback mechanism in intake control, then it is understandable that horses have reduced intakes of straw.

2.4 Silages

The use of ensiled forage is becoming increasingly popular for horse and pony feeding, and recent research has examined the relationship between the dry matter content of different silages, and the VDMI of these materials (Table 4).

The intakes of ponies fed limited amounts (1.65kgDM/100kgW) of grass-derived products, hay, haylage, big-bale silage and clamp silage were significantly ($p<0.05$) different (Moore-Colyer and Longland, 2000). Similar, but lower, intakes of both long and short chopped big bale silage have been reported elsewhere (Morrow, Moore-Colyer and Longland, 1999). It appears that the type of forage ensiled in bales has a major impact on intake. For example, Hale and Moore-Colyer (2001) measured the voluntary intakes of big-bale grass and big-bale red clover silages, compared with grass hay. Ponies consumed significantly ($p<0.05$) more red clover silage than hay; grass silage intakes were intermediate. The authors argued that maintenance of constant bodyweight implied some degree of intake regulation although the short duration of the trial makes this conclusion uncertain. Low intakes of clamp grass silage (<0.50 of hay intake) by horses have been previously reported by others (McLean, Afzalzadeh, Bates, Mayes and Hovell, 1995). These low intakes were associated with significantly ($p<0.01$) longer MRT compared to a hay diet; 51.7h compared with 36.8h using either chromium-mordanted hay or C32 alkane (McLean, 2001). Since physical regulation of intake appears to be unimportant in the horse, dry matter content of the forage cannot account for these measured differences although intake of maize silage has been shown to fall as dry matter content falls (Agabriel, Trillaud-Geyl, Martin-Rosset and Jussiaux, 1982). However, the nature of the conservation process is usually less good in low dry matter silages; fermentation characteristics of clamp silage have long been known to affect its intake by ruminants (for example see McCullough, 1966) and perhaps they also affect the DMI of horses. *Ad libitum* feeding of maize silage (DM:315g/kg) to horses resulted in very low intakes (40.6g/kg$W^{.75}$) and considerable refusals although conservation quality was satisfactory (Martin-Rosset and Dulphy, 1987). This contrasted with *ad libitum* hay intakes in the same study of 99.1gDM/kg$W^{.75}$.

Table 4. Relationship between silage type, dry matter content and voluntary dry matter intake of horses.

Silage type	Horse type	DM Content (g/kg)	Voluntary dry matter intake	Reference
Hay		922	62.9	
Haylage	Limit fed	676	79.2	Moore-Colyer and Longland (2000)
Big-bale silage	ponies	500	74.6	
Clamp silage		337	38.8	
Big-bale silage, long chop and short chop			63gDM/kg$W^{0.75}$	Morrow et al., (1999)
Big-bale grass		371	6.13 kgDM/d	
Big-bale red clover	Ponies	268	7.2 kgDM/d	Hale and Moore-Colyer (2001)
Grass hay		852	5.5 kgDM/d	

2.5 Concentrates

Horses are rarely allowed *ad libitum* access to concentrated feed. One study was reported (Cuddeford and Hyslop, 1996) in which ponies were offered a high fibre feed (NDF:418; CP:166) and consumed between 76 and 137 (mean 104) gDM/kgW$^{.75}$. On average the animals consumed in excess of three times their calculated digestible energy (DE) requirement, thereby indicating that equids fail to regulate their energy intake, at least in the short term. A more recent study (Argo, Fuller and Cox, 2001) compared the DE intakes of pony mares offered *ad libitum* access to the same complete diet in a pelleted or chaff form. Mean DE intakes of chaff and pellets increased ($p<0.01$) to attain maxima of 1.15 (0.11) and 1.76 (0.25) MJ/kgW$^{.75}$ on days 25 and 26 respectively. During this period of time intakes of chaff-fed animals were only 0.73 ($p<0.001$) of pellet DE intake and during a second period (days 35 to 63), it was 0.79 ($p<0.01$). By the end of this second period, the digestibilities of measured parameters significantly declined ($p<0.001$) for both diets; GE:-0.16 and NDF:-0.28 and as a consequence, chaff DE intake was reduced to 0.68 (0.07) MJ/kgW$^{.75}$. Although condition score and average daily gain increased over the first 4 weeks, growth and appetite returned to near maintenance values within 9 weeks. The authors concluded that nutritional characterisation of *ad libitum* diets must account for physiological adaptation that in this case, took some 35 days; Ralston (1992) abandoned an *ad libitum* experiment after 5 weeks possibly just when intakes might have stabilised or reduced. In view of the fact that most Latin Square experiments utilise 21-day periods, intake data obtained from *ad libitum* feeding experiments under these circumstances would be of questionable validity.

2.6 Conclusion

It would appear that many of the data reported have been from short-term experiments using classical experimental designs (e.g. Latin squares) that do not allow sufficient time for physiological adaptation to enable true measures of intake. However, it seems clear, that in equids, there is not the strong relationship, measured in ruminants, between NDF content and intake. Perhaps this is simply due to the absence of a metering device in the horse that is analogous to the reticulo-omasal orifice. Alternatively, perhaps the horse responds to the "bulkiness" of the food on offer. Kyriazakis and Emmans (1995) proposed that in pigs, water-holding capacity (WHC) limited the intake of "bulky" foods rather than fibre content *per se*. Tsaras, Kyriazakis and Emmans (1998) tested the proposal that WHC of a food was an adequate descriptor of its "bulk" and concluded that it accounts for the effects of different foods on voluntary food intake of pigs. In contrast, CF, ADF and NDF of feeds were inadequate in this respect. In view of the fact that sugar beet pulp has been shown to depress voluntary food intake by horses (Hyslop, Roy and Cuddeford, 1998; Hyslop and Cuddeford, 1999), perhaps the WHC of horse feeds should be assessed. This could then be related to intake rather than continue to seek a relationship between fibre content *per se,* and intake. It is clear that equids are more sensitive to the feel, smell and taste of their food than are ruminants and thus, oro-pharyngeal monitoring is more important in this species. Horse feed manufacturers recognise the importance of the organoleptic qualities of their products and this is apparent by their liberal use of syrups/molasses etc., to metaphorically "sweeten the pill".

3. Influence of breed and physiological status on intake

A diet of 0.85 meadow hay and 0.15 concentrate was fed *ad libitum* to dry, pregnant and lactating heavy horse (Comtois and Breton) breeds; their respective DMI's were 117, 113 and 162g/kgW$^{.75}$ (Martin-Rosset, Doreau, Boulot and Miraglia, 1990). In the same study, light horse geldings consumed 100gDM/kgW$^{.75}$; this was significantly less ($p<0.02$) than that of the dry mares. The voluntary food intakes of heavy breeds and lactating mares were respectively significantly greater than light breeds and non- lactating mares.

4. Effect of processing forage on its intake by horses

The physical form of the forage is important because it affects the rate at which the horse can consume its feed; the quantity of fibre (for example g NDF/kg DM) *per se* is meaningless in this context. Grass can be presented to a performance horse in at least five forms; fresh, ensiled, artificially dehydrated, sun-cured or dried, ground and then pelleted. The rate at which dry matter is consumed will be lowest with the fresh grass and highest with the pellets because the concentration of DM (g DM/kg) in the latter will be about five times greater than it is in the grass. An early experiment (Haenlein, Holdren and Yoon, 1966) demonstrated that three different physical forms of alfalfa hay (loose, wafered and pelleted) were consumed in different amounts. Whilst the three different diets were similar in chemical composition, they differed significantly in density and in mean particle size. Horses consumed 0.17 more wafers and 0.24 more pellets than loose hay. The CF of the pellets was significantly ($p<0.01$) less well digested than that of the loose hay presumably, reflecting a more rapid rate of passage through the gut. Todd *et al.*, (1995) obtained similar results when feeding different forms of alfalfa to horses. When alfalfa-based forages are fed *ad libitum,* the range of voluntary DMI's (gDM/kg$W^{0.75}$) reported in the literature are 75.3 to 122.0 for hays (Haenlein *et al.*, 1966; Cymbaluk, 1990; Crozier *et al.*, 1997; Dulphy *et al.*, 1997a; 1997b), 88.3 to 138.8 for dried wafers, cubes or pellets (Haenlein *et al.*, 1966; Cymbaluk, 1990; Todd *et al.*, 1995) and 100.0 to 155.0 for short-chopped, artificially dried material (Pearson *et al.*, 2001).

The rapid consumption of pelleted feed is often associated with the development of abnormal behaviours such as wood chewing (Haenlein *et al.*, 1966) and possibly, the onset of disease (Frape, 1998). Although the rate of consumption can be affected by modifying the physical form of forage with a resultant increase in total voluntary food intake, this is not always the case. For example, *ad libitum* provision of short-chop, dehydrated grass or traditional grass hay, both made from the same, second cut perennial ryegrass sward cut on the same day, resulted in similar intakes by ponies (Hyslop *et al.*, 1998). Earlier Gallagher, Hintz and Schryver (1984) had shown that chopping hay into a chaff form did not influence the digestibility of OM or ADF. Furthermore, Morrow *et al.*, (1999) measured no difference in nutrient digestibility or digesta passage rate when ponies were fed hay, either in long (18cm) or short-chop (5.3cm) form. These authors also showed that long and short-chop (29.3 and 6.8cm respectively) forms of big bale silage did not differ in these respects. Thus, the extent of physical treatment of forage will affect whether or not DM intake changes and whether digestibility parameters remain the same. Forages produced for admixture with concentrates, compounds or cereals are normally sold as "chops" or "chaffs"; the nutrient digestibilty and digesta passage rates for these materials should be the same as if the unprocessed forage were fed.

5. Conclusion

The animal's daily rate of nutrient extraction from forages is a product of the animal's daily food intake and the digestibility of the ingested forage. The latter will depend on fibre content and the rate of passage of forage through the GIT. The strategy adopted by hind-gut fermenters is to eat relatively more than ruminants (Janis, 1976), especially of high fibre foods, because, without a selective delaying mechanism for large particles, digesta passes quickly through the fermentation zone (caecum and colon). Equids are capable of extracting more nutrients per day from *ad libitum* forage diets than bovids (Duncan, Foose, Gordon, Gakahu and Lloyd, 1990) although perhaps the daily energetic costs of the extra grazing (~5h longer) outweigh the benefits. It is clear that the maximisation of DMI is critical to the adequate supply of nutrients to the horse. However, experiments that have measured straw intakes suggest that the model proposed for the horse does not hold true. Ponies fed *ad libitum* artificially dehydrated lucerne or oat straw consumed respectively, 155.0 or 94.7gDM/kg$W^{0.75}$ and when restricted to 0.70 of *ad libitum intake*, the equivalent figures were 70.2 or 67.5gDM/kg$W^{0.75}$ (Pearson *et al.*, 2001). Both the *ad libitum* intakes of lucerne and oat straw exceeded previously published values (see above) although this could have been a seasonal effect, resulting from the extended photoperiod during the summer months of the experiment. This would agree with the observations of Fuller, Argo and Cox (1998) that ponies had higher digestible energy intakes on long 'day-lengths' than on short 'day-lengths'. Apart from the apparent seasonal effect, ponies consumed less straw than lucerne and chromium-fibre MRT's were longer for the straw diets when compared to the respective lucerne diets (Pearson *et al.*, 2001). Was the longer MRT of oat straw a reflection of its lower intake, lower digestibility, slower rate of emptying from the colon or lower CP content? Was the lower VDMI of oat straw relative to lucerne, a reflection of its higher NDF content (715 vs. 443g/kgDM), lower OM digestibility (0.44 vs. 0.58), longer MRT of chromium-fibre (*ad libitum*, 31.5 vs. 21.3; restricted, 36.0 vs. 30.5h), lower CP content (38.8 vs. 146g/kgDM) or just greater faecal bulk? These questions remain to be answered.

References

Agabriel, J., Trillaud-Geyl, C., Martin-Rosset, M. and Jussiaux, M., 1982. Utilisation de l'ensilage de mais par le poulain de boucherie. Bulletin Technical CRZV Theix, INRA, 49: 5-13.

Aiken, G.E., Potter, G.D., Conrad, B.E. and Evans, J.W., 1989. Voluntary intake and digestion of Coastal Bermuda grass hay by yearling and mature horses. Equine Veterinary Science, 9: 262-264.

Argo, C.McG., Fuller, Z. and Cox, J.E., 2001. Digestible energy intakes, growth and feeding behaviour of pony mares offered *ad libitum* access to a complete diet in a pelleted or chaff-based form. Proceedings of the 17th Equine Nutrition and Physiology Symposium, Kentucky, USA. p.171-173.

Crozier, J.A., Allen, V.G., Jack, N.E., Fontenot, J.P. and Cochran, M.A., 1997. Digestibility, apparent mineral absorption and voluntary intake by horses fed alfalfa, tall fescue and caucasian bluestem. Journal of Animal Science, 75: 1651-1658.

Cymbaluk, N.F., 1990. Comparison of forage digestion by cattle and horses. Canadian Journal of Animal Science, 70: 601-610.

Cuddeford, D., and Hyslop, J.J., 1996. Intake and digestibility of a high fibre concentrate offered *ad libitum* to ponies and donkies. Proceedings of the 47th Annual Meeting of the EAAP, Lillehammer, Norway, p.296(a).

Dulphy, J.P., Martin-Rosset, W., Dubroeucq, H. and Jailler, M., 1997b. Evaluation of voluntary intake of forage trough-fed to light horses. Comparison with sheep. Factors of variation and prediction. Livestock Production Science, 52: 97-104.

Dulphy, J.P., Martin-Rosset, W., Dubroeucq, H., Ballet, J.M., Detour, A. and Jailler, M., 1997a. Compared feeding patterns in *ad libitum* intake of dry forages by horses and sheep. Livestock Production Science, 52: 49-56.

Duncan, P., Foose, T.J., Gordon, I.J., Gakahu, C.G. and lloyd, M., 1990. Comparative nutrient extraction from forages by grazing bovids and equids: a test of the nutritional model of equid/bovid competition and coexistence. Oecologia, 84: 411-418.

Frape, D., 1998. Equine Nutrition and Feeding. Second edition, Blackwell Science Ltd., Oxford, UK.

Frape, D.L., Tuck, M.G., Sutcliffe, N.H. and Jones, D.B., 1982. The use of inert markers in the measurement of the digestibility of cubed concentrate and of hay given in several proportions to the pony, horse and white rhinoceros (*Diceros simus*). Comparative Biochemistry and Physiology, 72A: 77-83.

Friend, M.A. and Nash, D., 2000. Pasture intake by grazing horses. RIRDC Publication No 00/. Project No UCS-22A. Rural Industries Research and Development Corporation, Australia.

Forbes, J.M., 1988. Metabolic aspects of the regulation of voluntary food intake and appetite. In: Nutrition Research Reviews 1. Cambridge University Press, Cambridge.

Fuller, Z., Cox, J.E. and Argo C.McG., 1998. Photoperiodic entrainment of seasonal changes in appetite and growth in pony colts. In: Proceedings of the British Society for Animal Science. P133.

Gallagher, J.R., Hintz, H. and Schryver, H.F., 1984. A nutritional evaluation of chopped hay for equines. Animal Production in Australia, 15: 349-352.

Gibbs, J. and Smith, G.P., 1978. The gut and preabsorptive satiety. Acta-Hepato-Gastroenterology, 25: 413-416.

Grace, N.D., Gee, E.K., Firth, E.C. and Shaw, H.L., 2002. Digestible energy intake, dry matter digestibility and mineral status of grazing New Zealand thoroughbred yearlings. New Zealand Veterinary Journal, 49, (In press).

Haenlein, G.F., Holdren, R.D. and Yoon, Y.M., 1966. Comparative responses of horses and sheep to different physical forms of alfalfa. Journal of Animal Science, 25: 740-743.

Hale, C.E. and Moore-Colyer, M.J.S., 2001. Voluntary food intake and apparent digestibilities of hay, big-bale grass silage and red clover silage by ponies. Proceedings of the 17th Equine Nutrition and Physiology Symposium, Kentucky, USA. p.468-469.

Hyslop, J.J. and Calder, S., 2001. Voluntary intake and apparent digestibility in ponies offered alfalfa based forages *ad libitum*. Proceedings of the British Society of Animal Science, p. 90.

Hyslop, J.J. and Cuddeford, D., 1999. Soaked unmolassed sugar beet pulp as a partial forage replacer in equine diets when ponies are offered grass hay *ad libitum*. Proceedings of the British Society of Animal Science, p.140.

Hyslop, J.J., Bayley, A., Tomlinson, A.L. and Cuddeford, D., 1998. Voluntary feed intake and apparent digestibility *in vivo* in ponies given *ad libitum* access to dehydrated grass or hay harvested from the same grass crop. Proceedings of the British Society of Animal Science, p.131.

Hyslop, J.J., Roy, S. and Cuddeford, D., 1998. *Ad libitum* sugar beet pulp as the major fibre source in equine diets when ponies are offered a restricted amount of mature grass hay. Proceedings of the British Society of Animal Science, p. 132.

Hyslop, J.J., Tomlinson, A.L., Bayley, A. and Cuddeford, D., 1998. Voluntary feed intake and apparent digestibility *in vivo* in ponies offered a mature threshed grass hay *ad libitum*. Proceedings of the British Society of Animal Science, p.130.

Janis, C.M., 1976. The evolutionary strategy of the Equidae and the origins of rumen and caecal digestion. Evolution, 30: 757-774.

Kyriazakis, I. and Emmans, G.C., 1995. The voluntary food intake of pigs given feeds based on wheat bran, dried citrus pulp and grass meal, in relation to measurements of food bulk. British Journal of Nutrition, 73: 191-207.

Laut, J.E., Houpt, K.A., Hintz, H.F. and Houpt, T.R., 1985. The effects of caloric dilution on meal patterns and feed intake in ponies. Physiology and Behaviour, 35: 549-554.

Lawrence, A.C.St., Lawrence, L.M. and Coleman, R.J., 2001. Using an empirical equation to predict voluntary intake of grass hays by mature equids. Proceedings of the 17th Equine Nutrition and Physiology Symposium, Kentucky, USA. p.99-100.

Martin-Rosset, W. and Dulphy, J.P., 1987. Digestibility interactions between forages and concentrates in horses: influence of feeding level-comparison with sheep. Livestock Production Science, 17, 263-276.

Martin-Rosset, W., Doreau, M., Boulot, S. and Miraglia, N., 1990. Influence of level of feeding and physiological state on diet digestibility in light and heavy breed horses. Livestock Production Science, 25: 257-264.

McCullough, M.E., 1966. The nutritive value of silage as influenced by silage fermentation and ration supplementation. Proceedings of the 10th International Grassland Conference, Helsinki, p.581.

McLean, B.M.L., 2001. Estimating digesta passage rate of forage based diets in horses using N-alkanes. Proceedings of the 17th Equine Nutrition and Physiology Symposium, Kentucky, USA. p.192-194.

McLean, B.M.L., Afzalzadeh, A., Bates, L., Mayes, R.W. and Hovell, F.D. DeB., 1995. Voluntary intake, digestibility and rate of passage of a hay and a silage fed to horses and to cattle. Animal Science, 60, 555.

McMeniman, N.P., 2000. Nutrition of grazing broodmares, their foals and young horses. RIRDC Publication No 00/28. Project No UQ-45A. Rural Industries Research and Development Corporation, Australia.
Minson, D.J., 1990. Forage in Ruminant Nutrition. Academic Press, New York.
Moore-Colyer, M.J.S. and Longland, A.C., 2000. Intakes and *in vivo* apparent digestibilities of four types of conserved grass forage by ponies. Animal Science, 71: 527-534.
Morrow, H.J., Moore-Colyer, M.J.S. and Longland, A.C., 1999. The apparent digestibilities and rates of passage of two chop lengths of big bale silage and hay in ponies. Proceedings of the British Society of Animal Science, BSAS, P.O. Box 3, Penicuik, Midlothian, EH26 0RZ, UK. p.142.
Pearson, R.A., Archibald, R.F. and Muirhead, R.H., 2001. The effect of forage quality and level of feeding on digestibility and gastrintestinal transit time of oat straw and alfalfa given to ponies and donkeys. British Journal of Nutrition, 85: 599-606.
Pearson, R.A. and Merritt, J.B., 1991. Intake, digestion and gastrointestinal transit time in resting donkeys and ponies and exercised donkeys given *ad libitum* hay and straw. Equine Veterinary Journal, 23: 339-343.
Ralston, S.L., 1984. Controls of feeding in horses. Journal of Animal Science, 59: 1354-1361.
Ralston, S.L., 1992. Regulation of feed intake in the horse in relation to gastrointestinal disease. Pferdeheilkunde, p.15-18.
Ralston, S.L. and Baile, C.A., 1982a. Plasma glucose and insulin concentrations and feeding behaviour in ponies. Journal of Animal Science, 54: 1132-1137.
Ralston, S.L. and Baile, C.A., 1982b. Gastrointestinal stimuli in the control of feed intake in ponies. Journal of Animal Science, 55: 243-253.
Ralston, S.L. and Baile, C.A., 1983. Effects of intragastric xylose, sodium chloride and corn oil on feeding behaviour of ponies. Journal of Animal Science, 56: 302-308.
Ralston, S.L., Freeman, D.E. and Baile, C.A., 1983. Volatile fatty acids and the role of the large intestine in the control of feed intake in ponies. Journal of Animal Science, 57: 815-820.
Todd, L., Sauer, W.C., Christopherson, R.J., Coleman, R.J. and Caine, W.R., 1995. The effect of feeding different forms of alfalfa on nutrient digestibility and voluntary intake in mature horses. Journal of Animal Physiology and Animal Nutrition, 73: 1-8.
Tsaras, L.N., Kyriazakis, I. and Emmans, G.C., 1998. The prediction of the voluntary food intake of pigs on poor quality foods. Animal Science, 66: 713-723.

European systems used for evaluating the protein requirements of performance horses

Evaluation and expression of protein allowances and protein value of feeds in the MADC system for the performance horse

W. Martin-Rosset[1] *and J.L. Tisserand*[2]

[1]*Department of Animal Husbandry & Nutrition, INRA - Center of Research of Clermont-Ferrand / Theix, 63122 Saint-Genès-Champanelle, France*
[2]*Etablissement National d'Enseignement Supérieur Agronomique (ENESAD) de Dijon, BP 87999, 26 Bd Docteur Petitjean, 21079 Dijon, France*

1. Introduction

MADC system was performed by INRA in France. This system provide sets of tables that give protein value of the feeds and the nutrient requirements of the horses respectively (INRA, 1984). Both are expressed according to the same feed evaluation system MADC for protein. The goals of this system in relation with the UFC system stated for energy (cf. Martin-Rosset and Vermorel's report in the issue) is to allow:
1) an accurate comparison of the nutritive value of feedstuffs;
2) the formulation of well balanced rations to achieve a production goal;
3) the prediction of the animal performance when amount and quality of rations are known

The validity of the MADC system was tested through many feeding trials using mares, growing horses and working horses to state the new french feeding standards (Martin-Rosset et al., 1994). This system was updated in the years nineties by the same INRA group on the bases of further experiments carried out on nitrogen digestion namely (Tisserand and Martin-Rosset, 1996).

This system is official feeding standards in France (INRA, 1990) and it is used in an increasing number of European countries with or without local adaptations (Miraglia and Olivieri, 1990; Staun, 1990; Smolders, 1990; Austbø, 1996). But there is still an increasing demand for new developments of this original MADC concept and their subsequent methods and tools for predicting protein allowances.

This paper will give the main figures used for stating the MADC system 1) nitrogen metabolism and nitrogen expenditures of the performance horse (young and adult) 2) evaluation of nitrogen value of feedstuffs used to meet the requirements 3) evaluation and expression of protein recommanded allowances

2. Nitrogen metabolism, expenditures and requirements

2.1 Nitrogen metabolism

The total protein content range between 17-19% of the body weight in the horse as in the other animal species. 55% Of the protein are in the muscles, 30% are in the conjonctive tissues whatever 7-8% are in the digestive tract or in the liver There are only 3% of protein in the blood.
All these proteins are continuously degraded or (and) synthetized according to different turn over as to whether the protein locations. Protein turn over of the muscular fibers range daily between 1 to 2% which is much longer than the turn over of protein in the digestive wall tract, liver, included enzymes and hormones, but faster than in the conjonctive tissues.

Protein balance of muscles is positive only during the amino acids (AA) absorption phase. Out of this period the protein requirements of digestive tract, liver... is much higher and the muscles provide AA such as alanine, glycine. Those two AA account for 30-40% of amino nitrogen supplied by peripheric tissues. These AA are the form for transporting nitrogen and carbon from the muscle to the liver, the digestive wall tract and the kidneys.The blood account for only 1% of total free AA. But variation in the quality of dietary proteins is reflected by the variations in the proportions of free AA in the blood (Reitnour and Salisbury, 1976; Rogers et al., 1981; Cabrera and Tisserand, 1995).

AA which are not used for synthesis are catabolised in the liver. Catabolised AA provided either carbon skeletton for producing glucose through neoglucogenis, fatty acids, ketones bodies, or amino group for synthesing urea (namely alanine and glutamine). This AA oxidative catabolism provides energy to the horse which is to be determined. In ruminants it reaches 15p100 of energy expenditure at maintenance(Lindsay, 1980-1982: Oldham and Lindsay, 1983). But the amount of catabolised AA depends on the energy supply to the liver and on the urea supply to the kidney. Catabolism increases too when the absorbed AA are unbalanced and when the protein intake is lower than the requirement and finally if catabolism is higher than synthesis.

2.1.1 Maintenance

At maintenance 15 g/kg $BW^{0.75}$ would be synthetised daily in the horse e.g. 1600 g for 500 kg body weight. The horse would synthetise 3 to 5 times more proteins than the AA intake as other herbivores species (Reeds and Harris, 1981). Most of the AA implemented for synthesis are provided by the own degradation of the body protein according to what is already known in other animals species (Millward et al., 1983).

2.1.2 Growth

In the growing horses protein synthesis is 2-3 times higher than in the adult. Synthesis for increasing body mass increase the synthesis devoted to the turn over as well. In addition the protein turn over is faster in the young horse than in the adult. As a result the total amount of proteins daily synthetised is far much higher than the amount of fixed proteins. The total amount of protein synthetised change in the same way as the amount which is fixed, thus as the daily gain. But it depends on nitrogen or (and) energy intake, both have additive effects (Reeds and Fuller, 1983).

2.1.3 Work

As early as we know Kellner pointed out that nitrogen catabolism increases in horses as far as the work rises (Kellner 1879, 1880, 1909) Later on von Liebig stated that muscle protein could provide fuel for muscle contraction. During working, protein synthesis in the muscles and in the digestive tract decreases but catabolism rises in the horse as in the human (Rennie et al., 1981; Millward et al., 1982; Booth and Watson, 1985). Using radioisotope labelled AA it has been demonstrated that when AA are used for energy the carbon skeleton is subjected to oxydative catabolism. Amino groups are transported from muscle to the liver where there are used either for non essential AA synthesis or excreted as urea. Transportation form of nitrogen is alanine for following transamination reaction amino groups are attached to pyruvate. In the liver nitrogen supplied by alanine is used to produce urea whereas the pyruvate is involved in neoglucogenesis. Plasma alanine concentration is known to increase during moderate exercise (Mc Keever et al., 1986; Miller and Lawrence, 1988; Esssen-Gustavsson et al., 1991; Miller-Graber et al., 1991a and 1991b). Plasma urea, creatine and uric acid increase following endurance race (Luke et al., 1980; Snow and al., 1982). Nitrogen catabolism carries on during several hours following the end of exercise as it is for energy with oxygen debt. Urea is mainly excreted by the sweat because renal excretion rate does not change during the exercise. From studies carried out in human (Young, 1986) branched AA could be oxydised to provide energy, namely leucine, isoleucine, valine. Training would reduce the AA catabolism during the exercise.

On the other hand, nitrogen retention would increase during exercise periods. It would rise at the begining of training as nitrogen intake increase as well with the increase of DM intake when rations are isoenergetic to maintain steady body weight (table 1). In the well trained horses the nitrogen balance would increase as far as nitrogen content rise where the DCP/DE of the diet is kept constant to maintain steady body weight (table 2). The nitrogen retention rate would rise faster than the increase of nitrogen intake. It could explain the development of muscular mass which has been measured by the increase of RNA concentration (Freeman et al., 1985a).

Amino groups provided by the AA catabolism, and ammonia which are absorbed in the digestive tract, are used for urea synthesis in the liver. Urea is excreted in the urine and in the digestive tract. Urea is hydrolysed in the digestive tract in ammonia which is either used for AA synthesis by microflora or reabsorbed if in excess. But there is no significant correlation between plasma urea concentration and urea degradation (Prior et al., 1974). Ammonia produced by further degradation of microbial proteins in the large intestine, is absorbed as well. Thus there is an entero-hepatic urea cycle in the horse as in the other herbivores which allows the animal to spare nitrogen

Table 1. Nitrogen balance in horses fed varying levels of nitrogen intake, (from Freeman et al., 1985a) (horses are offered an isoenergetic diet to keep constant body weight).

	Treatment			
Variable	1	2	3	4
Nitrogen content of diet (%)	7.3	7.6	11.6	13.6
Intake	102.4^{d}	114.9^{cd}	139.1^{c}	167.0^{b}
Fecal excretion	38.7	36.3	36.7	39.2
Urine elimination	29.3^{d}	38.0^{cd}	53.5^{bc}	72.9^{b}
Balance	34.4^{c}	40.6^{bc}	48.9^{bc}	54.9^{b}

[a] Minimum significant difference (P<.05)

[b, c, d] Means with different superscripts in same row differ (P<.05)

Table 2. Nitrogen balance in response to conditioning (from Freeman et al., 1985b) (horses are offered a diet with DCP constant fitted to keep constant body weigh) DE.

Variable	Treatment		
	1	2	3
Intake	81.8^{c}	120.8^{b}	105.3^{b}
Fecal excretion	25.2^{c}	44.0^{b}	30.5^{c}
Urine elimination	38.5	42.4	45.3
Balance	18.0^{c}	34.5^{b}	29.4^{bc}

[a] Minimum significant difference (P<.05)

[b;c] Means within same row with different superscripts differ (P<.05) and to supply nitrogen to microflora in the large intestine when nitrogen intake is too low (Houp and Houpt, 1971; Prior et al., 1974). 60% of urea produced would be excreted in the intestine of ponies fed with very low nitrogen diet, and 50% of this nitrogen would be recovered (Prior et al., 1974). Exogenous urea can be used by horse through this entero-hepatic cycle, but less efficiently than by ruminants (Slade et al., 1970; Houpt and Houpt, 1971; Hintz et al., 1972; Glade, 1984): 10 to 30% of this nitrogen would be recovered.

Under normal circumstances the whole absorbed ammonia is used mainly for urea synthesis but for the synthesis of AA as well if carbon skeletton is available through transamination pathway (Robinson and Slade, 1974).

2.2 Nitrogen expenditures and requirements

2.2.1 Maintenance

At maintenance urinary losses are estimated to be 128-165 mg/kgBW$^{0.75}$ (Hintz and Schryver, 1972; Prior et al., 1974; Meyer, 1983) whereas fecal losses would be 3 g/kg total dry matter intake (Meyer, 1983). Skin and sweat losses are evaluated to be 35 mg/kg BW$^{0.75}$ (Meyer, 1983) and 1g N/l (Winkel, 1977) respectively. Sweat losses would increase with dietary nitrogen intake when it is in excess to requirements (Eckersall et al., 1982).

2.2.2 Work

At work sweat losses increase and urine losses to a lesser extend as well. But the requirements rise too due to either the increase of the muscular mass mainly at the begining of training (Freeman et al., 1985b) or to enzymes and hemoglobines concentrations required by the metabolism of the exercising horse.

During endurance events where horse run 80 km at 18km/hour 2 to 3 mg of nitrogen losses / BW$^{0.75}$ / hour were measured in sweat by Snow et al., 1982. The losses rise with the nitrogen content of diet (Patterson et al., 1985, Miller-Graber et al., 1990) as the protein catabolism increase (Lucke et al., 1980, Snow et al., 1982). Sweat is the major route for urea excretion as the kidney excretion rate does not rise during the exercise. In a horse of 500 kg BW nitrogen losses in sweat could range daily 25-37 g during intense work as estimated by Meyer (1987).

The amount of nitrogen expenditure in exercising horse is not exactly known but there is a consensus to tell that nitrogen requirements would increase with regular work. In addition NRC (1989) and INRA (1984-1990) recommandations stated the same protein/energy ratio in the diet of working horse as in the diets of horse at maintenance. Graham-Thiers et al. (1999) have recently pointed out that there is a significant interaction between a high fat diet in combination with restricted protein fortified with lysine and threonine to improve quality of nitrogen turnover or (and) additionnal muscle development.

INRA stated that nitrogen expenditure increase more slowly than the energy expenditure referring to the work of Kellner (1909) and old recommendations drawn from feeding trials (cf. review of Olsson and Ruudverre, 1955). But nitrogen expenditure might increase more or less when body proteins are used to supply a lack of energy reserves or (and) intake as pointed out by the respiratory quotient (RQ) measured by Pagan et al. (1987) in exercising horse fed either with carbohydrates or protein diets (figures 1 and 2).

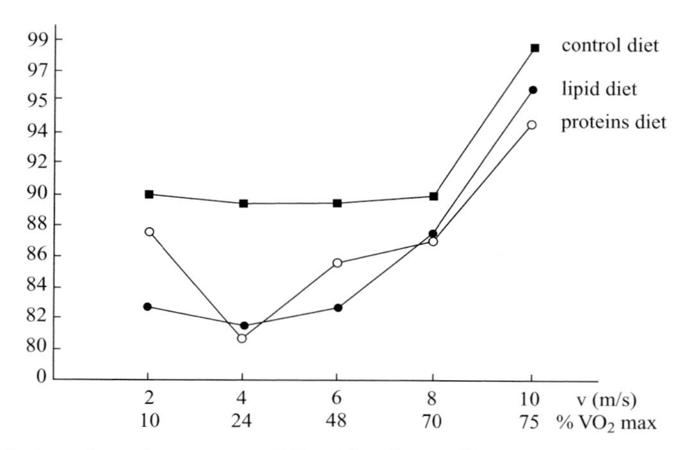

Figure 1. Variation of respiratory rate (RR) with velocity (from Pagan et al., 1987).

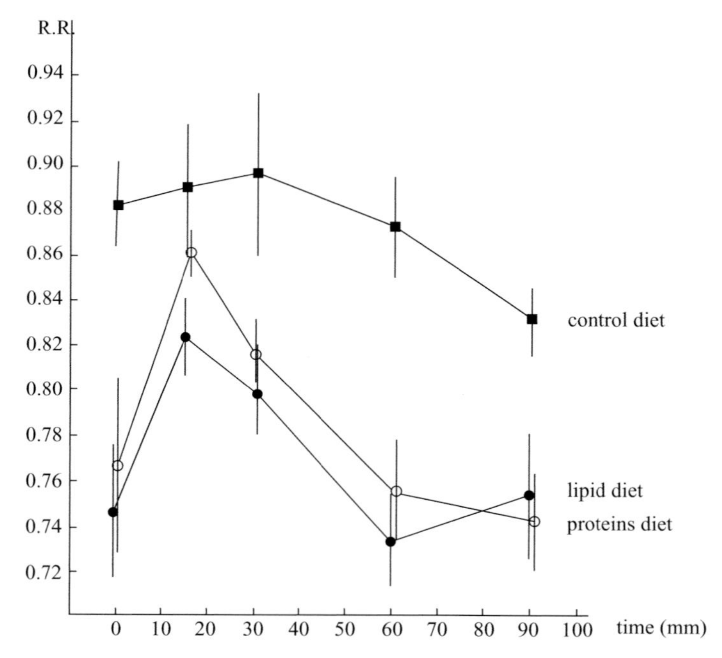

Figure 2. Variation of respiratory rate (RR) with duration at trot 300 m/mn (from Pagan et al., 1991).

2.2.3 Growth

In the young horse, the body composition varies with age as the proportions of the different tissues changes. Drawn from data obtained in heavy breeds the proportion of muscle decrases from 51 to 40 p100 as the relative growth coefficient (b) to empty body weight is b = 1.1 during the breeding period (with no exercise). But the proportion of adipose tissues rises from 8 to 10 p100 for relative growth coefficient reaches b = 2.1. Proportion of bone tissues decreases from 11 to 10 p100 as b = 0.7 (Martin-Rosset et al., 1983b). As a result chemical composition of empty body weight changes between weaning to 2.5 years of age (figure 3): proteins content decreases slightly from 22 to 20%. In addition protein content of live weight gain decreases from 25 to 20% when average daily gain (ADG) increases from 600 g to 1100 g (table 3).

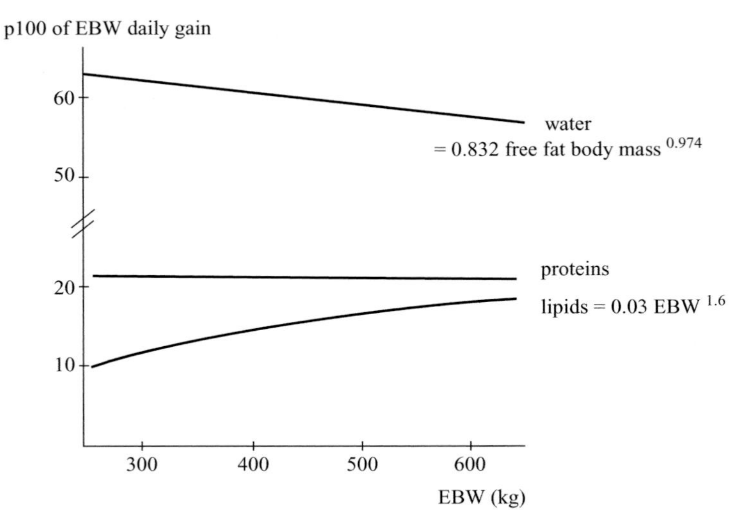

Figure 3. Evolution of chemical composition of Empty Body Weight (EBW) daily gain between 6 to 30 months (drawn from Agabriel et al., 1984).

From all the feeding trials carried out those last 3 decades in USA (Jarrige and Tisserand, 1984; Ott, 2001) two main conclusions can be drawn:

- daily gain increases with protein content of the diet but partially due to increase in dry matter intake as well.
- Quality of protein is of major concern namely lysine and threonine.

Nitrogen requirement for growth can be estimated by 1 kg of ADG above maintenance using the factorial method e.g. dividing fixed protein by metabolic efficiency rate of digestible protein (DP) for growth. The efficiency rate was stated to be 45 p100 (Jarrige and Tisserand, 1984). But due to the lack of measurement of the evolution in chemical composition of body weight and daily gain and of experimental trials designed namely to determine protein requirement in light breeds as for heavy breeds (Agabriel et al., 1984) the requirements were performed by INRA with global method by using data drawn from feeding trials conducted especially by INRA for that purpose (Agabriel et al., 1984, Bigot et al., 1987, Trillaud-Geyl et al., 1992).

A mathematic model similar to that used for energy was designed (table 4). In this model requirements depends on body weight as for maintenance and to daily gain not affected by an exponent as for energy because the variation in protein content of daily gain is rather low compared to lipids content variation (Agabriel et al., 1984). It must be pointed out that protein requirement for maintenance decreases from 3.5 g MADC/kg $BW^{0.75}$ before 1 year to 2.8 g MADC/kg $BW^{0.75}$ after 1 year which is the same as in the adult. Protein requirement of daily gain decreases nearly by 2 times between the two periods (in the model b = 450 vs 270) as well in accordance with variation in protein content of daily gain.

Table 3. Chemical composition of daily gain in yearling and long yearling of heavy breeds in different situations (drawn from Agabriel et al., 1984).

Type of animal	Daily gain of BW[1] g/d	Daily gain of EBW[1] g/d	Chemical composition of EBW[1] daily gain		Chemical composition of BW[1] daily gain		
			Lipids p.100	Protein p.100	Lipids p.100	Protein p.100	Energy Cal.
Yearling (6-12 months)							
1st trial[2]	1100	890	13	20.9	10.6	16.9	1890
2nd trial[3]	500	400	- 5.5	25.2	- 4.4	20.2	825[4]
	1000	800	11.3	21.1	9.0	16.9	1720
	1390	1100	15.9	19.7	12.6	15.6	2060
Long Yearling (12-18 months)							
Growth during the prior winter							
• slow		950	8-11	21-22			
• moderate		840	2-6	23-24			

[1] BW = Body Weight; EBW = Empty Body Weight

[2] Average values observed in yearlings fed with the same diet: anatomical composition was measured by dissection of half carcass

[3] Referenced values obtained when comparing yearlings affected by different feeding levels: anatomical composition was predicted from anatomical dissection of the 14th rib according to Martin-Rosset et al., 1985.

[4] Lipids content was considered to be 0

Table 4. Requirements for growth (from Martin-Rosset et al., 1994).

Energy: relationship between daily energy intake and live weight and growth in young horses of light breeds $UFC/day/kgW^{.75} = a+bG^{1.4}$			Protein: relationship between daily protein intake and live weight and growth in young horses of light breeds $g\ MADC/day = aW^{.75} + bG$		
Ages (months)	a[1]	b	Ages (months)	a[1]	b
6-2	0.0602	0.0183	6-12	3.5	450
18-24	0.0594	0.0252	12-24	2.8	270
30-36	0.0594	0.0252	30-36	2.8	270

[1]a: Coefficient for maintenance
G: average daily gain (kg/day)
1.4. Allometric coefficient of lipids in total body weight relatively to empty body weight

Data from Agabriel et al., 1984 & INRA unpublished results

Lysine and threonine are the two limiting AA as stated from the work of Breuer and Golden (1971) Ott et al. (1979, 1981 and 1983), Saastamoinen et al. (1993) and from the work of Graham et al. (1994) respectively. But feed protein quality is of less importance as the growth potential decreases with age and the proportion of hay in the diet increases simultaneously.

3. Evaluation, expression and prediction of the protein value of feedstuffs

3.1 Bases of the system

The Horse Digestible Crude Protein (Matières Azotées Digestibles Cheval: MADC, in French) System is based on two concepts (Jarrige and Tisserand, 1984; Tisserand and Martin-Rosset, 1996).

- Nitrogen value of feedstuffs depends on the amount of amino acids (AA) truly provided by the feedstuffs,
- The amount of AA provided by feedstuffs depends on the site of digestion in the digestive tract: small intestine vs large intestine

Non protein nitrogen (NPN) may account for 10 to 30% of total nitrogen in forages, depending on the type of forages graminea vs legumes, the vegetative stage and the method for conservation of hay or silage. In concentrate NPN is low.

The true N digestibility of nitrogen from the small intestine was estimated from the studies conducted with markers in slaughtered or ileal fistulated animals (cf. reviews of Jarrige and Tisserand, 1984; Martin-Rosset et al., 1994; Cudderford, 1997; see Potter's report in this issue) or performed recently with mobile nylon bag technique (MNBT) in fistulated horses in France at INRA (Cordelet, 1990; Macheboeuf et al., 1996) or in Scotland at the University of Edimburgh (Moore-Coolyer et al., 1998).

True N digestibility in the small intestine range form 30-40% for hays to 60-75% for mixed diet or 50 to 80% for cakes as measured namely by the Texas A-M group in USA when the MADC system was performed by INRA in 1984.

As a result true N digestibility in the small intestine was estimated by INRA in the MADC system to be:

- 30-45% for hays
- 60% for dehydrated alfafa
- 60-70% for grass
- 70-80% for concentrates

The true N digestibility of feeds reaching the large intestine measured in slaughtered equines, in fistulated equines (cf. reviews of Jarrige and Tisserand, 1984; Martin-Rosset et al., 1994; Cudderford, 1997; or original work: Glade, 1983-1984; Potter et al., 1992; and report in this issue) ranges between 75-90% for forages and concentrates (cereals and cakes).

Feed proteins (and endogenous proteins) are degraded partially in the large intestine as AA, peptides and ammonia and resynthetised to microbial proteins according to available energy and the type of nitrogen consumed (Robinson and Slade, 1974; Meyer, 1983; Martin-Rosset et al., 1994). Microbial proteins thereafter provided free AA and ammonia. It was assumed by INRA that no more than 10-30% of nitrogen in the large intestine would be absorbed as AA and peptides from the works conducted on the efficiency of AA absorption in the large intestine (Slade et al.,

1971; Goodbee and Slade, 1972; Wysocki and Baker, 1975). It is in accordance with what were determined in pigs (Rerat, 1981) and in ruminants (INRA, 1978).

Finally, fecal nitrogen is composed of indigestible feed nitrogen mostly bound to fiber (so called acid detergent insoluble nitrogen or ADIN): 5% on average (Nicoletti et al., 1980), endogenous nitrogen (3 g N/kg TDMI - Total Dry Matter Intake (Meyer, 1983)) and microbial protein nitrogen (50-60% of total N in feces (Meyer et al., 1993)) endogenous N + bacterial N would account for 88% of total N fecal (Nicoletti et al., 1980). Amount of soluble nitrogen is rather low: 5 to 8% of total N fecal (Nicoletti et al., 1980).

From the above considerations the protein value of feedstuffs for the horse is referred to as the sum of feed and microbial AA absorbed in the small and large intestines, respectively and expressed in Horse Digestible Crude Protein (MADC).

The attempt to evaluate amount of absorbable AA in the digestive tract point out that DCP overestimate the value of forage expressed in MADC by 10 to 30% (table 5).

As a result MAD content of the main groupe of forages is calculated by reducing their DCP content by:
- 10% for green forages
- 15% for hays and dehydrated forages
- 30% for good quality grass silages

or multiplying DCP content respectively by a factor k which is 0.90, 0.85, 0.70 for the forages listed previously.

MADC value is only a quantitative evaluation of the AA content of feedstuffs. The expression has to be refined for specific requirements lysine and threonine for growth.

For concentrates MADC content account for their DCP content as feed nitrogen is mainly digested in the small intestine, namely grains and feeds. For by products with heavy cell wall content, MADC content might be corrected by ADF content (Martin-Rosset et al., in progress).

This expression of nitrogen value in MADC allow to improve the comparison of feeds and to substitute themselves when formulting the diets. The correcting factor K will be improved as far as we will know any more about amount of AA which are absorbed.

3.2 Test of the validity of the MADC system

Different figures of the MADC system were assumed by INRA in 1984. Then validity was tested by different workers during the year nineties.

3.2.1 Digestibility in the small intestine

A proportion of feed protein is excreted in the feces: the Non Digestible Crude Protein (NDCP) which is related to the CP content (Robinson and Slade, 1970; Martin-Rosset et al., 1984). The NDCP decreases linearly as proportion of concentrate in the diet increases from 0 to 60% (Martin-Rosset and Dulphy, 1987) for protein of concentrates are namely digested in the small intestine.

$NDCP = 0.285\ C - 78.0 \qquad R^2 = 0.366^{**}$

Table 5. Assessment of the amount of absorbable intestinal amino-acids (expressed in AIA) provided by some feedstuffs, Comparison between forages and concentrates (in g/kg DM)[a] (from Jarrige and Tisserand 1984).

Feedstuffs	Crude protein		Small intestine			Large intestine				Total tract	
	Total g	Non-aminated g	Entry g	True digestibility	AIAA g	Entry g[1]	True digestibility	AIAA %[2]	AIAA g	MADC g	DCP g
Rich concentrates (crude fiber 8%)	180	9	171	0.85	145	26	0.90	10	2	147	148
								30	7	152	
				0.75	128	43		10	4	132	
								30	12	140	
Green grass at early grazing stage	180	18	162	0.70	113	49	0.80	10	4	117	123
								30	12	125	
				0.60	97	65		10	5	102	
								30	16	113	
Barley-corn mixture	110	5	105	0.85	89	16	0.90	10	1	90	90
								30	4	93	
				0.75	79	26		10	2	81	
								30	7	86	
Grass hay (at heading)	110	11	99	0.50	50	49	0.75	10	4	54	65
								30	11	61	
				0.40	40	59		10	4	44	
								30	13	53	
Grass silage	110	28	82	0.50	41	41	0.75	10	3	11	65
								30	9	50	
				0.40	33	49		10	4	37	
								30	11	44	

[1] Entry: in gr of aminated nitrogen provided by feeds

[2] Percentage of alimentary proteins absorbed as amino acids and peptides

AIAA: Absorbable Intestinal Amino Acid

True digestibility of feed protein was estimated to be 40% and 70% for hays and concentrates (cereals and cakes) respectively (Gibbs et al., 1988; Potter et al., 1992; Farley et al., 1995) and 50-60% for mixed diet (Almeida et al., 1999; Coleman et al., 2001) in ileal fistulated ponies. For mixed diet there would be no effect of protein levels in diet on the precaecal digestibility of AA (Almeida et al., 1999) which is unconsistent with the previous data (cf. review of Jarrige and Tisserand, 1984; Martin-Rosset et al., 1994) but in accordance with recent data of Macheboeuf et al. (1995) observed with forage diets (table 6).

Recently INRA has determined true digestibillity of feed protein in horses with a mobile nylon bag technique (Macheboeuf et al., 1995-1996). True N digestibility reach 60%, 60-85% and 80-90% for hays, cereals and issues, and cakes respectively (Macheboeuf et al., 2003; Martin-Rosset et al., in progress). For hays true N digestibility does not seem to be highly affected by cell wall content

Table 6. N digestibility of hays in the small intestine and in the total tract in horses mesured by the mobile nylon bag technique (from Macheboeuf et al., 1995).

Hay		1	2	3	4	5	6	7
Composition								
N(% DM)		0.76	1.03	1.50	1.55	1.56	2.46	2.63
N-ndf/N (%)		40.7	50.1	50.3	59.1	50.3	53.1	62.3
Total tract								
N digestibility (%)	MNBT	65.2	61.7	68.5	68.2	75.4	83.9	79.8
	In vivo	46.6	42.0	54.5	60.1	56.7	64.7	64.6
N true digestibility (%)	MNBT	74.9	79.6	79.6	82.1	83.6	91.3	88.4
	In vivo	79.4	76.5	81.2	86.2	83.7	89.6	88.4
Precaecal N digestion (NMBT)								
% N intake		67.3	62.4	62.3	60.7	65.6	65.4	60.9
% digestible N intake		103.2	101.2	90.9	89.0	87.0	78.0	76.3
% truly digestible N intake		89.9	78.5	78.2	73.9	78.5	71.7	68.9

(figure 4) For concentrates there is a relevant relationship between the true total N digestibility calculated in 1984 (INRA tables) and the N digestibillity measured in the small intestine (figure 5).

The heavy weight of small intestine for digestion of feed proteins is confirmed. True digestibility coefficient of hays, grains and cakes reach 50%, 75% and 85% respectively.

3.2.2 Digestibility in the large intestine

True digestion coefficients of feed nitrogen measured in slaughtered equines (Glade, 1983 and 1984), in ileal fistulated ponies (Gibbs et al., 1983-1988; Potter et al., 1992; Farley et al., 1995) and with mobile nylon bag introduced through a caecal fistula in ponies (Cordelet, 1990) or reintroduced throught the caecal fistula after having being introduced previously in the stomach through a probe and collected at the end of samll intestine (Macheboeuf et al., 1995), range between 79-90% for forages and concentrates (cereals and cakes). For very poor forages: straw, nitrogen digestion depends on energy and nitrogen supplementation of the diet (Glade, 1984).

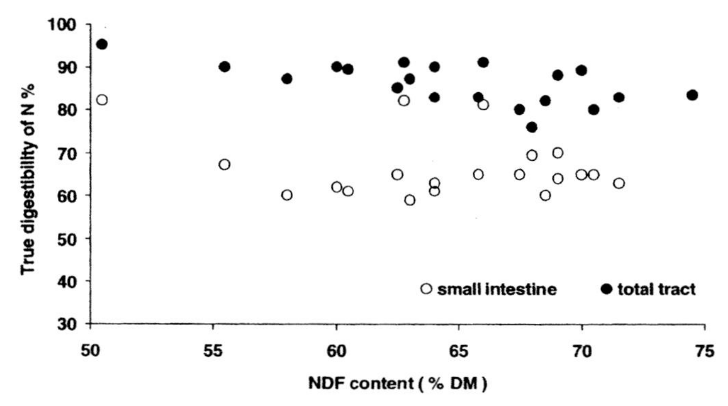

Figure 4. Effect of NDF content on true digestibility of nitrogen of hays in the small intestine (from Martin-Rosset et al., in progress).

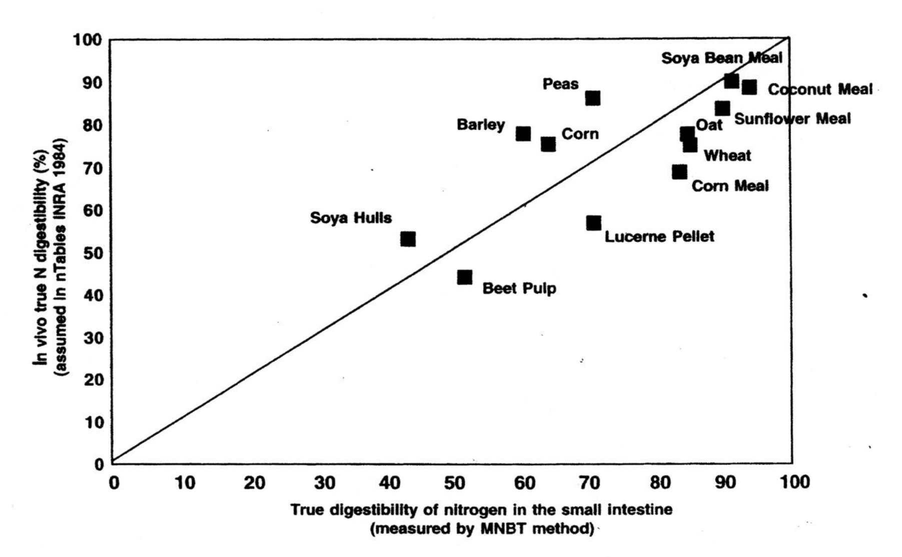

Figure 5. Relation between in vivo digestibilities drawn from INRA tables and precaecal ND for concentrates (from Martin-Rosset et al., in progress).

Feed nitrogen digested in the large intestine is mainly used for synthesis of microbial protein. Microbial protein content of feces decreases tremendously in horses fed mixed pelleted diets (lucerne + cereals) after resection of the colon (Bertone et al., 1989).

3.2.3 Absorption of amino acids

Serum protein levels in ponies bypassed for Jejunum and ileum is significantly lower than in control ponies fed mixed diet (Frank et al., 1983). In the small intestine, digestion of feed nitrogen might be affected by the schedule of feeding-time of the different feeds of the diets: concentrates VS forages. Plasma concentration of AA measured in the jugular vein of ponies fed a straw-corn and soya bean meal diet is significantly higher between 3 to 6 hours after feeding when the nitrogen supplement is fed two hours later on the forage meals (Cabrera and Tisserand, 1995).

Caecal bacteria are known to be able to use AA for synthetising their own protein (Baruc et al., 1983) and the growth of proteolytic microbial population would be stimulated by dietary nitrogen provided by soja supplementation (Julliand and Tisserand, 1992). But there own nitrogen requirement ar not yet determined (Maczulack et al., 1983). The caecal bacteria are able to produce some extracellular AA (Baruc et al., 1983). Using isotopic technique and labelled cysteine infused into the caecum or into the colon or horses Mc Meniman et al., 1987 pointed on that only 1 to 6% of the plasma cysteine was of microbial origin.

Homoarginine was used by Schmitz et al. (1990) as a modele to study AA absorption from the large intestine as homoarginine is detected only in traces in blood. There was no significant homoarginine detectable in blood after infusion of homoarginine into the caecum. Using the technique of overdosing five different AA: threonine, valine, methionine, phenylalanine and lysine infused into the colon of fistulated pony Tisserand et al., (in progress) confirm that there is no increase of AA plasma concentration in the colic vein (figure 6).

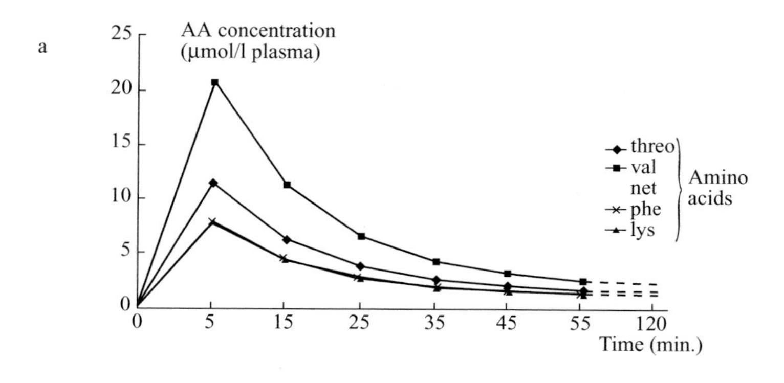

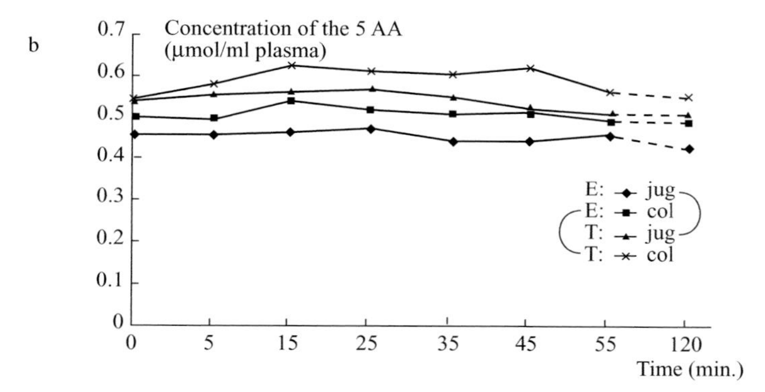

Figure 6. a. Effect of overdose of AA infused into the colon on plasma AA concentration in the colic vein of fistulated pony (from Tisserand et al., unpublished).
b. Comparison of the average plasma concentration of the 5AA in the jugular vein (jug) and in the colic vein (col) after (E) or without (T) overdose of the 5 AA infused in the colon (from Tisserand et al., unpublished).

As a result there is no active AA absorption in the large intestine although microbial protein can be digested by microbial enzymes (Baruc et al., 1983). Passive diffusion of AA across the large intestine wall might occur to explain slight appearance of isotopes (N_{15} or C_{14}) in the blood observed by Slade et al. (1971) and Wysocki and Baker (1975). But it is quite controversed by in vitro observation of Bochroder et al. (1992 and 1994) who pointed out the impermeability of the colon mucosa to AA.

It can be concluded that the microbial AA synthetised within the large intestine do not significantly contribute to the AA supply of equine.

3.3 Prediction of MADC value of feedstuffs

The nitrogen value of feeds can be predicted in the MADC system either from feed tables or calculated from the chemical composition of feeds by using the appropriate relationship (Martin-Rosset et al., 1994).

3.3.1 Feed tables

Feed tables were set up for horses by INRA. The chemical composition was drawn from tables for ruminants in the case of forages (INRA, 1978) and in the case of concentrates and by products from tables for monogastric (INRA, 1984) or (and) ruminants (INRA, 1978).

The DCP content of all forages were estimated using the relationship between DCP and CP content of forages studied in digestion trials conducted in horses by INRA (Martin-Rosset et al., 1984) and drawn from the litterature (table 7). The DCP content were corrected by the appropriate factor K (table 8) to be expressed in MADC.

Table 7. Relationship between DCP content (g/kg DM) and CP content (g/kg DM) in forages (from Martin-Rosset et al., 1984-1994).

	n	Relationships	RSD	R
Fresh forages				
Natural grassland, grasses	14	DCP = - 27.33 + 0.8614 CP	± 7.7	0.967[1]
		DCP = - 74.52 + 0.9568 CP + 0.1167 CF	± 6.3	0.980[2]
Hays				
Natural grassland grasses	47	DCP = - 25.96 + 0.8357 CP	± 7.1	0.968[3]
Legumes	25	DCP = - 29.95 + 0.8673 CP	± 9.2	0.933[4]
All forages	72	DCP = - 27.57 + 0.8441 CP	± 8.6	0.964[5]

Table 8. Calculation of MADC value of feedstuffs with INRA system (from Martin-Rosset et al., 1984-1994).

MADC = DCP X k

k = 1 for concentrates
k = 0.90 for green forages
k = 0.85 for hays and dehydrated forages
k = 0.80 for straws and their by products with high lignin content
k = 0.70 for good grass silages

The MADC value of forages can be predicted directly with the tables when the botanical characteristics and the conditions at harvest are well known.

The CP digestibilities of concentrates come partially from digestibility experiments carried out by INRA (Martin-Rosset et al., 1984) and others in horses fed forages supplemented with more than 25% of concentrates. The digestibility was also drawn from pigs tables when the crude fiber content was less than 15% (peas, cakes) or extrapolated from pigs and ruminants tables in some cases (dehydrated potatoe pulp, linseed meal, palm kernel meal, maïze bran). These CP digestibillities of concentrates will be improved in the next future when revising INRA tables with data obtained by Wolter et al. (1979-1982) in ponies as it has been pointed out that digestibililty coefficients are not significantly different from those measured in horses (Vermorel et al., 1997) and from data of Martin-Rosset et al. (1990-1995) and Smolders et al. (1990).

3.3.2 Calculation from chemical composition

The MADC value of *forages* in the horse is the DCP content corrected for the proportion of DCP which does not supply AA. MADC content (g/kg DM) is calculated from DCP (g/kg DM) content (table 8) multiplied by a correction factor k which depends on the groupe of forages (table 8).

The DCP content of forages is closely linked to the CP content (table 7). In the case of green forages the improvement is not highly significant by introducing CF in prediction equation. The relationships are not so different between green forages and hays. And calcuation of equations for each different botanical groupe does not improve accuracy of DCP prediction. As a result, equations (1) and (5) might be better to use.

The MADC content of *concentrates* is not different of DCP content. Due to the lack of enough experimental data in 1984, no correction was calculated for DCP content of raw materials namely byproducts where high content in cell wall should restrict protein digestion when compared to grains and needs. It might be introduced a reduction which should be proportionnal to cell wall content expressed in crude fiber, ADF or ADL in the next future thanks to recent data obtained by INRA (Martin-Rosset et al., in progress). By the time the DCP content (g/kg DM) of cereals and by products can be predicted with the following relationship when CP is expressed in g/kg DM

$DCP = 4.94 + 0.8533\ CP$
$RSD \pm 7.7 \qquad R = 0.931 \qquad N = 23$

For the other concentrates the DCP content must be drawn from the tables.

3.4. Discussion and prospect

In the MADC system, nitrogen value of feedstuffs in horses is linked to CP content (and NPN/N ratio), to digestibility of CP digested either in the small intestine or in the large intestine.

Total digestibility of CP has been extensively measured in equine for forages and to a lesser extend for concentrates in France in the years 1980's (Wolter et al., Martin-Rosset et al.) and more recently in the Netherlands in the years 1990' (Smolders et al.).

Proportion of CP digested in the small and large intestine is now much more well known thanks to experiments carried out with fistulated equines in the USA (Potter et al., 1982-1995) and in Europe (Meyer et al., Wolter et al., Tisserand et al., Martin-Rosset et al., Cudderford et al.). Recent studies of brazilian or american workers with ileal fistulated horses and by INRA with MNBT method support the coefficient of true N digestibilities in the small intestine stated in the MADC system by INRA in 1984.

AA requirements are mainly supplied by AA absorbed in the small intestine when horses are fed a high proportions of concentrates. At the same DCP content, concentrates provide 20 to 40% more AA than forages.

The difference between forages and concentrates might be reduced as forage provide some essential AA and nitrogen sources, AA and/or ammonia to microbial population in the large intestine for synthesising microbial protein.

As the AA absorption in the large intestine should be considered very negligible, the MADC system should account in the future for any amount of AA (and ammonia) which are used by microflora to satisfy its own nitrogen requirements in respect to amount of available energy (Glade, 1984; Reitnour, 1979-1980) but with no respect to organic nitrogen sources (Julliand and Tisserand, 1992). Bacteria are known to be able to use AA (and NPN) for synthesizing (Baruc et al., 1983) their own protein at a rate estimated to reach 2.5 mg N/g DM/h in the caecum content (Slade et al., 1973).

As the AA absorption in the large intestine should be considered very negligible The different fraction of nitrogen in the fèces which are representative of nitrogen digestion and metabolism have been estimated: microbial proteins accounts for 50 to 60% nitrogen in the feces (Meyer, 1983), soluble nitrogen content of feces is low: 5 to 8% of total fecal N % DM (Nicoletti et al., 1980), endogenous nitrogen in the feces has been estimated from a large range of diets to be 3 g/kg DM (Meyer, 1983) and the endogenous nitrogen losses in the urine would reach 339 mg/kg $BW^{.75}$ for horse offered a mixed diet (Almeida et al., 1999).

What could be the evolution expected at short and long term in the future ?
More accurate true digestibilities of the protein provided by different type of forages due to botanic families legumes vs graminea, stage at harvest, and of different concentrates (raw materials): grains, seed and their by products should be provided at short time thank to the data recently obtained over a large range of forages (n=21) and concentrates (n=16) by INRA using the MNBT method (Martin-Rosset et al., in progress). For raw materials a relationship between DCP value and cell wall content might be performed to improve the prediction of MADC value.

The recent data obtained in AA digestibilities in the small intestine equine offered mixed diet by Almeida et al. (1999) pointed out a new fascinating long term challenge to express the nitrogen value of feedstuffs in AA content truly digested. If we compare equines to other animals such as pigs (or even ruminant such as dairy cow now) nitrogen requirements are expressed routinely in AA for pigs. The protein of ideal composition (e.g. AA proportions and EAA balanced proportions is always requested in pigs to optimise the efficiency rate of conversion as some relationships between EAA are stated now (INRA, 1988; NRC, 1999).

The lack of these information namely in growing horses (and mares) and to a lesser extend in exercising horses provides us an insight into some new challenges to refine the protein and AA requirements of the horse. But the improvment provided by this valuable approach will be relevant when ileal flux of AA will be performed for a large range of diets to weight the amount of AA supplied and when these data will be supported by long term feeding trials conducted with producing horses as well.

Increase in the knowledge of microbial protein synthesis in the large intestine should be the second key point to improve the accuracy of the MADC system.

Since the initial proposal of MADC system by INRA in 1984, microbial ecosystem of the large intestine is now considered to be namely an energy supplier for the host and a nitrogen supplier to itself through the ammonia-urea entero hepatic cycle and N extracted from dietary N bound to cell walls. As a result efficiency of protein microbial synthesis, ammonia production and absorption should be evaluated. The efficiency of these processes would depend on residual CP content and composition of dietary CP after enzymatic digestion in the small intestine, degradability (DT) of residual CP content of ileal digesta, amount and composition of fermentable organic matter (FOM) available and finally synchronisation of the availability of energy and nitrogen components to optimise the growth and the enzymatic activities of the microbial ecosystem. Promising work has been done in the years 1990's by Cordelet 1990 and then by Julliand 1996. Such approach should go on to estimate nitrogen requirement of microbial ecosystem. These nitrogen requirements might be not so far to the amount of AA estimated to be recovered in the large intestine (10-30% digestible N) in the scope of MADC system (INRA, 1984) ? Such new knowledges would allow to improve the MADC system: MADC value of feedstuffs would take into account for the AA requirements of the host and the nitrogen requirements of the microbial ecosystem.

Thus expression of nitrogen value in MADC is still up to date as it allows the integration of the most recent knowledge. Feeds can be easily compared each other and they can be substitued themselves for calculating balanced diet. But the system has to be refined for accounting particular AA requirement other than lysine and threonine in growing horses and mares.

4. Evaluation and expression of protein requirements and recommanded allowances

4.1 Definitions and methods for determination

In France, nutrient requirements and allowances are clearly distinguished. The requirements stand for physiological expenditure of horses for maintenance, growth and exercise (cf. I). The requirements are covered by the nutrients of the ration and by the body reserves when the amount of nutrients supplied is inadequate. The nutrient allowances represent the amount of the nutrients provided by the ration. A recommended allowance is the amount of nutrients which should be supplied to horses to achieve a desirable level of performance allowed by their potential. The animals are assumed to be in good health, well managed and housed during the winter period. These should be considered as optimum allowances, which cover at least the requirements. Exceptions are:

- *growing horses* bred for school-riding or hacking where limited growth is assumed during the winter period but a compensatory growth period is expected during the subsequent summer period to achieve an optimum body weight at late breacking (figure 7)
- *Exercising* horses where a moderate and controlled used of body reserves is assumed at short term (a few days) during the training period to avoid physiopathalogic disorders related to large variation in workload and subsequent daily nutrient intake.

The allowance can be estimated either by a factorial method from metabolic data and/or by feeding experiments according to the physiological function. With the factorial method, amount of proteins fixed or exported is divided by the metabolic efficiencies of the digestible crude protein (DCP) which are specific to the physiological function where these efficiencies are known. With the feeding method, the allowances are determined by long-term feeding trials (and nitrogen balances) conducted with a high number of animals. In these experiments, nitrogen intakes are related to the true performances.

4.2 Protein requirements and recommanded allowances

In the horse, as in other farm animals, a distinction between maintenance and production requirements has been made, although overall metabolism is influenced by variations in animal expenditures.

4.2.1 Maintenance

On the basis of the nitrogen balance set up by Slade et al. (1970), Hintz & Schryver (1972) and Prior et al. (1974), maintenance requirements have been estimated to be 2.7 g DCP (digestible crude protein) kg $BW^{0.75}$ which is the requirement stated by NRC (1978). Due to the lack of french

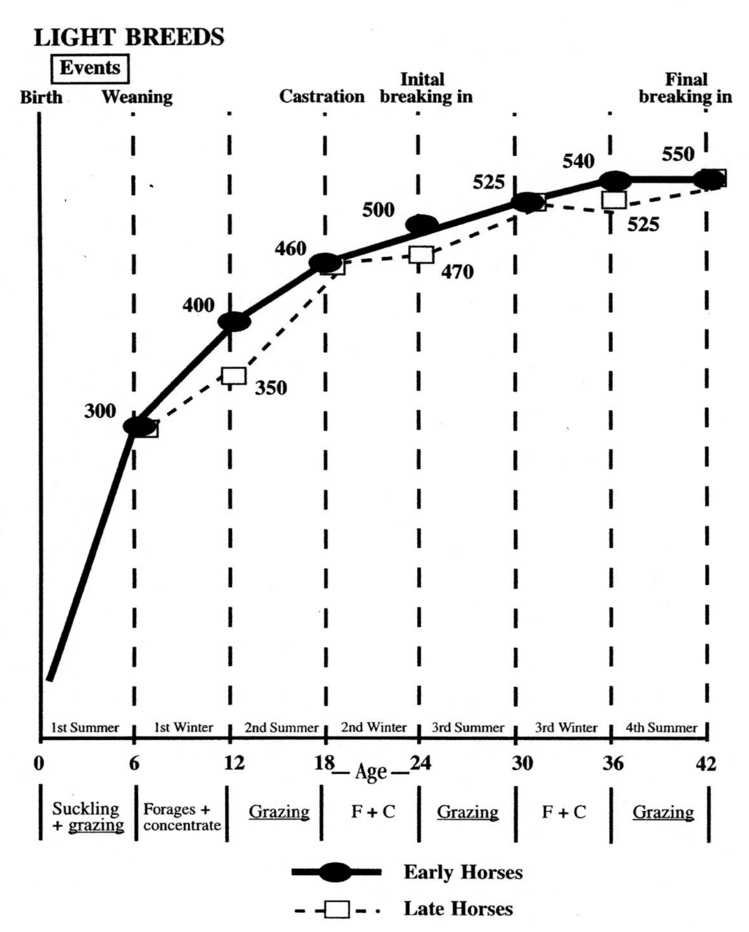

Figure 7. Growth curve and management of young sport horses (selle français or anglo-arabe) established from INRA long term feeding experiments (from INRA 1990).

data nitrogen requirements were stated to be 2.8 g MADC/kg $BW^{0.75}$ (INRA, 1984). It is close to the former requirements stated by Olsson and Ruudvere (1955). A a result amount of feeds allowances (e.g. dry matter intake to fit the requirements) is 10 to 15 p100 higher than those calculated from NRC (1978) as far as the DCP content of forage was decreased by 10 to 20 p100 with MADC system. (INRA, 1984; Jarrige and Tisserand, 1984). Daily allowances reach 295 g MADC for horses weighing 500kg. However, they are lower than those calculated with factorial method (Meyer, 1983) as this author took into account the possibilities of storing proteins.

All the feeding trials, digestion studies and nitrogen balances carried out show that the AA composition of the common diets for adults horses at maintenance is of no importance and that NPN (urea particularly) can be successfully used by the horse if the fermentable energy supply in the large intestine is sufficient.

4.2.2 Work

For work, protein expenses are unknown. They could increase more than energy expenses in relation to intensity and length of work if energy supply is not sufficient to prevent body protein mobilization (Kellner, 1909). Thus, there is some reason to relate protein and energy supply for work as for protein synthesis where the protein gain is positively related to the protein and energy contents of the diet (cf. I). A supply of 60 to 70 g MADC/UFC e.g. 30 g MADC/Mcal NE beyond maintenance requirements seems satisfactory for the adult horse at work. MADC recommanded allowances have been stated by INRA using this ratio (table 9). As a result for a 500 kgBW horse exercised 2 hours per day, daily MADC requirements would increase from 370 g to 620g according to work intensity (table 9). If we assume for this horse offered a 50/60 hay-concentrate diet to supply total nutrient requirements that protein apparent digestibility is about 65%, daily CP requirements would vary from 450 to 950 e.g. between 1.0 to 1.9 g CP/kg BW. For most human athletes 1.2 to 1.5 g CP/kg BW are suggested (Friedman and Lemond, 1989; Lemond, 1991). If we consider that protein sources consummed by human are likely of much higher quality and digestibility, the INRA recommandations are more comparable.
The relevance of higher protein diet offered to exercising adult to support changes in body composition such as increased muscle or lean body mass is not stated in horses (as in humans). This feeding practice is based on the assumption that lean body mass increase with training. In fact lean body mass percentage might rise sometimes for the body fat content would decrease simultaneously whereas there is not change in absolute lean body mass.

Table 9. Recommended daily energy (UFC or Mcal NE) and nitrogen (MADC) allowances for exercising sport and leisure horses of light breed (500 kg mature liveweight) (INRA 1990).

Use	Daily allowances[1]							Daily feed* (kg DM **)
	UFC (Mcal)	NE (Mcal)	MADC (g)	Ca (g)	P (g)	MG (g)	Na (g)	
Maintenance:								
Horse at rest	4.2	9.73	295	25	15	7	12	7.0-8.5
Work								
Very light[2, 4]	5.4	11.88	370	28	16	8	22	8.5-9.5
Light[2, 4]	6.9	15.18	470	30	18	9	37	9.5-11.5
Moderate[2, 4]	7.9	17.38	540	35	19	10	47	10.5-13.5
Intense[3]	7.2	15.95	490	35	19	10	40	10.0-12.0

* The lower values are used with high proportion of concentrate in the diet and the higher with hay-based diet

** DM: dry matter

[1] These recommendations are suggested for geldings and mares.0.4 UFC or 0.88 Mcal NE and 30 g MADC are added daily for stallions

[2] We considered two hours of daily work (mean observed in riding school)

[3] We considered one hour of daily work

[4] For short outside riding, very light and light work intensities are considered for one and two hours of exercise, respectively. For medium (2 to 4 hours) and long (> 4 hours) outside riding, light and moderate work intensities are considered

Protein supplementation above 1.5 g /CP.kg BW has probably no significant benefit for horses (Miller-Lawrence, 1988; Miller-Graber et al., 1991; Pagan et al., 1987) as for human (Wilmore and Freund Beau, 1984; Lemon et al., 1992).

In addition several studies suggest that diets containing excessive level of protein may be detrimental to equine performance. Increase in sweating, higher heart rates and urea plasma concentration and ultimately reduction of velocity would have be measured in endurance horse (Slade et al., 1975) but in contrast Glade (1984) and Hintz et al. (1980) did not observe any significant effect. The excess of protein could increase water intake (Meyer and Pferdekamp, 1980) and blood ammonia concentration as far as urea flux into the digestive tract rises (Schmidt et al., 1982) and ammonia production by muscles cellular increases too (Miller et al., 1985). Plasma ammonia concentration higher than 10 to 25 mg/l would make the horse excited (Hintz et al., 1970). Finally exercising horses offered daily high excess in crude protein, more than 3g CP/kg BW, compared to horses fed 2g CP/kg BW, excreted during exercise more nitrogen in sweat, had higher plasma urea concentration and orotic acid excretion. In the last case the rise in orotic acid excretion might suggest an overflow of urea cycle capacity (Miller-Graber et al., 1991).

Excess of protein would restrict the oxydative metabolism (Miller et al., 1985), muscle glycogen concentration and the RQ decrease as well (Pagan et al., 1987). But the effect on glycogen storage was less effective in the work of Miller-Graber et al., 1991. In horse fed very high protein diet, muscle and liver glycogen concentrations are reduced before exercise and muscle glycogen repletion post exercise is slowed (Satabin et al., 1989a, 1989b).

But AA balance of allowances in exercising adult horses might be reached as well. Comparing two diets: 7.5% CP diet with added lysine and threonine to 14.4% CP diet for working horse, Graham-Thiers et al. (1999) demonstrated the low protein AA supplemented diet had no adverse effect on the physiological parameters related to protein and energy metabolism. It can be concluded that the AA supplemented low protein diet met the requirements. On the other hand, extra AA provided by the high protein diet are deaminated as blood urea-N increased but blood ammonia levels were not affected. Blood lactate was depressed suggesting that glycogen was spared by extra supply of AA used straight away for energy metabolism. And ultimately blood alanine concentration was lower as well.

The administration of supplemental branched-chain AA before or (and) after training provided no measurable beneficial effect on energy metabolism in exercising horse (Stefanon et al., 2000; Casini et al., 2000). It can be concluded that AA requirements and allowances are not yet well designed in working horse.

4.2.3 Growing horse

In light breeds, protein requirements were calculated by using a mathematical model similar to that used for energy (table 4) as there were enough INRA feeding trials (Agabriel et al., 1984; Bigot et al., 1987; Trillaud-Geyl et al., 1992) designed to study effect of the CP content of the diet on average daily gain.

Two levels of allowances were suggested in growing horses as for energy considering the goal of production, genetic potential of the animal and the use (or not) of compensatory growth on pasture (table 10 and figure 7).

We have kept allowances suggested by NRC (1989) for lysine: 0.6% and 0.5% of total dry matter intake (TDMI) for weanling, yearling, two years old respectively. For threonine, Ott (2001) has

Table 10. Feeding standards for the growing horses - Recommended nutrient allowances. Horses of light breed - 500 kg mature body weight (INRA 1990).

Age (months)	Mean body weight during the period (kg)	Growth Level	Daily gain (g/d)	UFC (Mcal)	NE (Mcal)	MADC (g)	Ca (g)	P (g)	Mg (g)	Na (g)	Daily feed[1] kg/DM[2]
			Daily allowances								
Yealring	320	Optimal	700-800	5.5	12.10	590	39	22	10	12	5.5-8.0
(8-12)	280	Moderate	400-500	4.5	9.90	440	28	16	9	9	5.0-7.5
2 year old	470	Optimal	400-500	6.8	14.96	420	36	20	10	13	7.5-10.0
(20-24)	440	Moderate	150-200	6.0	13.20	330	28	16	9	12	7.0-10.0
3 year old	490	Optimal	150-250	6.5	14.30	330	30	18	10	12	8.0-11.0
(32-36)	470	Moderate	0-100	6.0	13.20	260	25	15	8	12	7.5-10.0

[1] The lower values are used with high proportion of concentrates in the diet and the higher values with hay based diet
[2] Dry matter

suggested 0.5 and 0.4% TDMI for the weanling and yearling respectively. For methionine experimental data are contradictory (Borton et al., 1973; Meakin et al., 1979). Tryptophan is not likely to be limiting as tryptophan content of horse feedstuffs is high (table 12). Feed protein quality is of less importance as the growth potential decrases with age and the proportion of hay in the diet increases simultaneously.

Concerning the long yearling and the 2 years old in training, a greater supply should be necessary to enable increases in muscular mass, in the concentrations of myoglobin and in enzymes responsible for muscular metabolism as well as to prevent anemia. For the human athlete, protein supply should be increased by 20% at the beginning of training and by 100% during intensive training (Willmore and Freund Beau, 1984). There is no evidence to increase the protein or AA supplementation to equine athlete over what it is recommended for human athletes (c.f. review of Lawrence, 1998).

4.2.4 Comparison of requirement expressed in MADC and CP

As far as the requirements suggested by NRC (1989) and INRA (1984-1990) are concerned and expressed in each system relative to maintenance as 100% bases, the NRC requirements seem to be lower than INRA requirements for nitrogen when comparing the relative differences between the two systems: from 0 to 26 p100 namely in the yearling (table 11).

5. Formulating diet to meet the requirements

5.1. Amount of protein

5.1.1 Adult horse

The protein requirements are always met in the working horses as far as the TDMI rises from 1.6 to 2.4 kg DM/100 kg BW (e.g. + 50 p100) to supply the energy requirements (INRA, 1990). There is no reason to increase highly MADC concentration of the diet in the working horse compared to

Table 11. Energy or nitrigen requirements (500 kg BW horse) expressed either in DE and CP system (NRC 1989) or in NE (or UFC) and MADC systems (INRA 1984-1990) related to maintenace in each system.

Systems	Energy			Nitrogen		
Animal	NRC	INRA	% NRC/INRA	NRC	INRA	%NRC/INRA
Mature horse						
• maintenance	100	100	100	100	100	100
Growing horse						
• yearling (12 months)						
– rapid growth	130	130	100	146	227	64
– moderate growth	115	107	107	130	169	76
• 2 years old (24 months) (not in training)						
– rapid growth	148	161	92	157	156	100
– moderate growth	113	142	80	120	122	98
Working horse						
• very light	125	128	98	125	137	91
• light	-	163	-	-	174	-
• moderate	150	187	80	150	200	75
• ± intense	200	172	116	200	182	110

resting horses. The MADC concentration of diet stated by INRA (1990) is: 68-70 g MADC/UFC (or 29 g MADC/Mcal NE) e.g. 38 to 45 g de MADC/kg DM (e.g. + 18 p100) as to whether the intensity of exercise (rest to intense) and according to TDMI recommanded intake. These recommandations are consistent with those of Meyer (1987). But NRC (1989) recommands crude protein (CP) concentration in the diet according to intensity of exercise: 40 g CP/Mcal DE e.g. 73 to 105 CP/kg DM (e.g. + 43 p100) as far as TDMI rises from 1.8 to 2.5 kg DM/100 kg BW (e.g. + 38 p100). In 1978, NRC recommanded 85 gDCP/kg TDMI. Discrepancies between INRA and NRC recommandations relatively to rest situation in both case might be due to: 1) diffrences in defining work intensity and as a result energy requirement and nitrogen requirement, 2) differences in TDMI/100 kg BW namely at rest and medium work.

In pratice, as far as proportion of grains in the diet increase to meet the energy requirement excess of nitrogen allowances rise due to high MADC/UFC ratio of most of the concentrates combined to MADC/UFC ratio of forages (table 12). Other energy sources such as vegetable oil or beet pulp might be used for formulating appropriate compounds feeds as experienced by Crandell et al. (2001).

5.1.2 Young horse

The protein requirements are rather easily met in the 2 year old exercising horse as far as the TDMI rises to meet the energy requirements as well (table 13).

Comparing non-working ***2 year old*** (470 kg BW) ***to yearling*** (320 kg BW) daily TDMI rises by 29 p100 (6.8 vs 8.8 kg TDMI) in the growing horses and comparing rest to moderate or intense

Table 12. Protein (MADC) Energy (UFC-NE or DE) ratio of the feedstuffs (kgDM) (from INRA Tables 1990).

Feedstuffs	g MADC/UFC	gMADC/Mcal NE*	g CP/Mcal DE
Soyabean meal	455	207	129
Sunflower meal	435	198	133
Linseed meal	351	160	109
Lupin sweet seed	318	113	88
Faba bean seed	250	113	88
Pea seed	190	87	67
Gluten feed	187	85	67
Wheat bran coarse	151	69	58
Soya hulls	114	52	55
Oat	97	45	34
Hays 1st cut (early heading)	88	40	46
Hays 1st cut (full heading)	82	37	44
Hays 1st cut (flowering)	77	35	43
Corn bran	81	37	35
Barley	79	31	33
Grass silage (prewilted: 30% DM)1st cut	72	27	32
INRA recommandations[1]	**68-70**	**27**	**26**
Corn	59	26	36
Beet pulp dehydrated	57	33	42
Corn silage (30% DM)	35	16	28
Corn starch	4	2	2
Cereals straw	0	0	22

[1] NE = 2200 kcal / kg fresh material for barley (INRA 1984-1994)

exercise in the working adult horse daily TDMI increase by 53 p100 on average (7.8 vs 12.0 kg TDMI). As a result TDMI would reach at least 2.2 kg DM/100 kg BW *in the 2 year old in training*. Simultaneously total protein requirements (growth + development of muscular mass + work) of exercising 2 year old might be 17% lower than in the yearling (table 13). MADC concentration of diet for the ***exercising 2 year old*** would be 65 g MADC/UFC, 62 g MADC/kg TDMI when at work (which is higher than that proposed for non working 2 year old in INRA recommandation 1990 (table 13). But these theoritical calculations are still questionable due to hypothesis done on increase in lean body mass and protein/energy requirements which are linked. There is some contradictory data in human which stress to be very carefull with nitrogen allowances.

In the ***yearling*** (320 kg BW) not exercised, the protein concentration would be higher 106 MADC/kg TDMI respectively as TDMI is rather limited 2.1 to 2.2 kg DM/100 kg BW.

Wilmore and Freund (1986) mention that in human weight lifters may have negative nitrogen balance during heavy training even fed with a high protein diet. The absolute lean body mass could be not affected by training whereas the proportion of lean body mass would increase for there would be simultaneously a reduction in body fat content. Ultimately the question concerning the amount of extra proteins (and energy) to be supplemented to increase muscular mass is still opened e.g. it has to be determined in respect of interaction between energy and protein on bone development as well (Martin-Rosset, 2001; Mc Ilwraith, 2001) to prevent bone disorders (table 14). Further research is needed.

Table 13. Protein allowances in young horses and adult.

		No exercise[1]	Light exercise[2] 1 h/d of walk
Yearling (12 months)	gMADC	590	(745) ? [3,5]
(6-12 mo)	UFC	5.5	7.3 [(4)]
320 kg BW	kg TDMI	6.75	7.00
	gMADC/kgTDMI	87	106
	gMADC/UFC	107	102
	kgTDMI/100kgBW	2.1	2.2
		No exercise[1]	Moderate exercise[2,6] 1 h/d
2 year old (24 months)	gMADC	420	618[3,5]
(18-24 mo)	UFC	6.8	(9.6) ?[4]
470 kg BW	kg TDMI	8.75	10.00
	gMADC/kgTDMI	48	62
	gMADC/UFC	62	65
	kgTDMI/100kgBW	1.9	2.1
		Rest[1]	Intense exercise[1,6] 1h/d
Adult	gMADC	295	490
500 kg BW	UFC	4.2	7.2
	kg TDMI	7.80	11.00
	gMADC/kgTDMI	38	45
	gMADC/UFC	70	68
	kgTDMI/100kgBW	1.6	2.3

[1] INRA 1990 recommandations

[2] Theoritical calculations

[3] Included:
- increase in protein requirement due to development of muscular mass
- increase in protein requirement due to exercise

[4] Included:
- increase in energy requirement due to increase in extra protein synthesis related to development in muscular mass
- increase in energy requirement due to exercise

[5] Increase in protein requirement for development of muscle (lean body mass): + 25% for the yearling; + 100% for the 2 year old. Protein / energy ratios are expected to be the same as for muscle growth at each age.

[6] Cf. INRA 1984-1990 recommandations for description of one hour of standardised work (Martin-Rosset et al., 1994)

MADC: Horse Digestible Crude Protein
UFC: Horse Feed Unit
TDMI: Total Dry Matter Intake
BW: Body weight
mo: months

( ) ?: theoritical calculation is questionnable and not ready straight away for formulating diets due to the hypothesis on protein turnover, N/E rations, additivity of protein metabolism events, variation in N retention due to N intake response to work conditinonning (cf. Freeman et al., 1985),. Comparing the MADC and UFC allowances stated for exercise vs no exercise situation. The truth is probably located between the two MADC and UFC values given in colum no exercise vs light or moderate exercise

Table 14. Effects of nitrogen or energy level in the diet on OCD appearance in the growing horse (from Savage - Mc Carthy - Jeffcott 1993).

	OCD[1]			
	n	Radio (Rx)	Post mortem	Histology
100% DE[2] CP[3]	12	0	1	2
129% DE (100% CP)	12	6	11	12
126% CP (100% DE)	6	0	1	4

[1] OCD: Osteochondrosis
[2] DE: Digestible energy
[3] Crude protein

The INRA recommandations range for growing horse (yearling - 2 year old) with no excercise from 107 g MADC/UFC to 62 g MADC/UFC and for growing with exercise from 102 g MADC/UFC to 65 g MADC/UFC:e.g. 106 to 62 g MADC/kg TDMI: x 1.7 times) for TDMI which range from 1.9 to 2.3 kg DM (INRA, 1990 and table 10).

These INRA recommandations are different from NRC recommandations for formulating diet. In NRC (1989) 45 g CP/Mcal DE are recommanded for the yearling, long yearling and 2 year old (e.g. 83 to 195 g CP/kg TDMI: x 2.3 times) as towether the age and in training or not (long yearling and 2 year old) and the recommanded TDMI ranges : from 2.1 to 2.5 kg DMI / 100 kg.

In the ***weanling*** (270 kg BW) the protein concentration of the diet should be very high 120-130 g MADC/kg TDMI as TDMI is restricted to 2.5 kg DM/100 kg BW.

In the ***nursing foal*** amount of milk and protein intake per kg of foal liveweight gain estimated by the dilution of deuteruim oxide as a marker foal body water and chemical analysis of milk respectively are at 1st and 2nd month of age: 10.6 kg of milk and 258 g of protein and 13.7 kg of milk and 292 g of protein (figures 9 and 10). Thereafter daily gain is depending on both milk, grass intake and eventually concentrate supplementation. Growth might be stimulated by concentrate supplementation to reach in the diet between 16% CP (Jordan and Myers, 1972) to 22% (Borton et al., 1973).

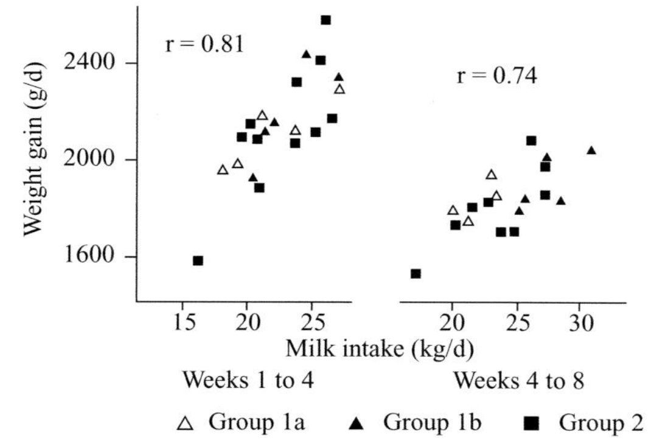

Figure 9. Relationship between foal milk intake and foal liveweight gain (mean and standard deviation) (from Doreau et al., 1986).

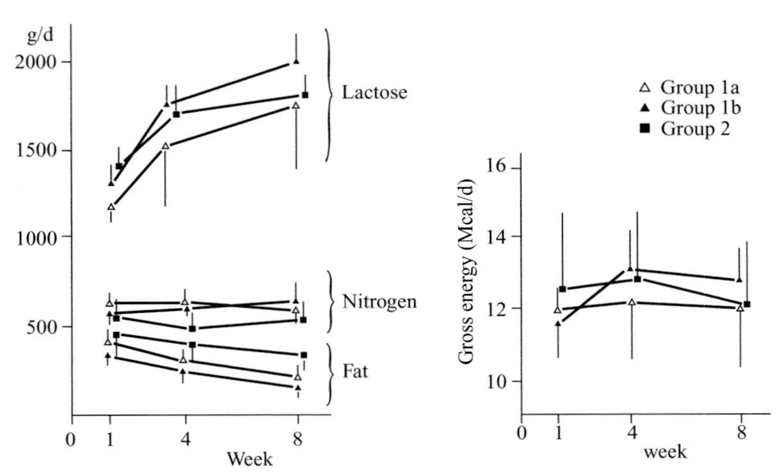

Figure 10. Quantity of foal nutrient intake (mean and standard deviation) (from Doreau et al., 1986).

5.1.3 Comparison of recommanded allowances in MADC (INRA, 1990) and CP (NRC, 1989) for formulating diet

The aim of any feeding system is to meet the requirement of the animals for type and level of production using available feeds. The nature, chemical composition and nutritive value of these feeds may vary with climatic and economic conditions. Ingestibility and palatability of feed, intake capacity of the animal and substitution rate between forages and concentrates must also be considered.

The differences between the NE and DE systems have been previously pointed out (cf. report of Martin-Rosset & Vermorel in this issue) and differences between MADC and DCP systems have been discussed as well c.f., paragraphe 2 in this report. Prediction of feed energy or nitrogen value in NE with regard to MADC and INRA systems has been described previously from a scientific point of view and primarily for the sake of application.

Energy and nitrogen requirements of different types of equines (growing or exercising horses) as well as the energy and nitrogen value of feeds and rations may vary between feeding systems.

As pointed out in the review of Hintz and Cymbaluk (1994), effect of environmental factors might be involved also, and added to the observed discrepancies which are acquainted to coefficients set up in the factorial method to perform the requirements of NRC primarily and of INRA partially. In the case of INRA recommendations, the procedure to implement allowances incorporates the impact of environmental factors because INRA allowances have been set up on feeding experiments designed and performed namely for this purpose whatever they are based or not on the requirements established from the factorial approach, depending on the physical function.

Cuddeford (1997) compared NRC and INRA requirements. For energy, comparison takes place on requirements expressed in DE in both NRC and INRA, assuming conversion rations from NE to DE drawn from INRA feed evaluation system. For nitrogen, Cudderford (1997) matched INRA requirement expressed in MADC to NRC requirement expressed in DCP, assuming digestion coefficient of CP drawn from NRC (1978). Conclusions are that NRC requirement would be slightly higher than INRA requirement for energy and for protein namely for growth.

As nutrients requirements of equine, as well as nutritive value of feeds and rations vary among feeding systems it is therefore, essential to evaluate whether total energy and protein requirements of equine of the different type of equines can be met by the same amount of feeds in balanced rations of the various feeding systems hereby NRC vs INRA.

Frape (1997) compared applications of DE (NRC, 1989) and NE (INRA, 1990) systems to the formulation of simple balanced daily rations based on grass hay, barley grain and extracted soyabean meal for a horse 500 kg at maturity in regard to energy and protein and with feed intakes, kg DM/day provided by NRC (1978). Total dry matter intakes (TDMI) for each type of animal are stated to be the same in the two feeding systems for a type of animal. As a result, the hay to concentrate ratios vary to match energy and protein requirements in each system. Dry matter intake for forage (DMIF) is lower with NRC system for all the type of equine, with the exception of exercising horse where it is higher. The discrispancies range between - 9 to - 24% (DMIF NRC-DMIF INRA/DMIF INRA) for breeding equine and and + 9 to + 19% for exercising equine respectively. Accounted some of outcome value in growing horse due to unrealistic hay concentrate-ratio (68 to 83%) the discrispancies range from - 8 to - 13% for breeding equine. The inconsistancy of difference between NRC and INRA may partially acquainted to difference in requirement between NRC and INRA. Description and as a result requirement of high and moderate work are different between the 2 systems (cf NRC, 1989 and INRA, 1990; Martin-Rosset et al., 1994). For example light work in NRC (1989) recommandations, seems to correspond to very light work in INRA (1990) recommandation.

As a result the appropriate procedure to compare the two systems that INRA proposes is as followed: requirements of each type of equine are provided in each system according to their performances level: DE, CP, TDMI for NRC (1989) and NE, MADC, TDMI for INRA (1990).

Good and poor (in some situations) quality hay based diets were tested. Forages were supplemented with barley and extracted soybean meal in appropriate proportions to meet the energy and protein requirements of the different type of equine depending on their performance level. The characteristics of the 4 feeds used are given in table 15.

The energy value (DE or NE per kg DM) and nitrogen value (CP or MADC, per kg DM) of each diet and the amount of feed required to meet energy and nitrogen requirements were computed in each energy and nitrogen system. In a first approach the hay-concentrate ratio was those proposed

Table 15. Chemical composition and nutritive value of feeds (for NRC/INRA system comparison).

Feeds	DM	/kg DM							
	g/kg	DE (Mcal)	NE (Mcal)	CF (g)	CP (g)	DCP (g)	MADC (g)	CP/DE	MADC/NE
Good grass hay (n° 62)[1]	850	2.34	1.34	333	102	59	50	44	37
Poor grass hay (n° 70)[1]	850	1.69	0.92	382	76	37	31	45	34
Barley grain (n° 120)[1]	860	3.56	2.55	54	117	92	92	33	36
Soyabean meal extracted 48-50 (N° 130)[1]	883	4.20	2.40	39	545	496	496	130	207

[1] Tables INRA 1984

by NRC (1989). Then, in a second step the hay concentrate ratio tested in in some situation were those proposed by INRA (1990).
For yearling (12 months) fed good hay supplemented with concentrate percentage proposed by NRC, TDMI differences between NRC and INRA balance rations are erratics ± 4 to 19% for rapid (0.750 kg/d) and moderates growth (0.450 kg/d) growth (table 16). But CP provided by balance good hay-concentrate ration calculated in the INRA system are - 16 to - 24% lower than the CP NRC requirements for moderate and rapid growth respectively (see table 16). Conversely the MADC provided by NRC balance hay-concentrate diet calculated in the NRC system are + 34 to + 35% higher than INRA requirements for moderate and rapid growth (table 16) respectively. And 60% concentrate for moderate growth suggested by NRC appears to be far too high in the INRA system: 40% could be more appropriate.
***For two year** old* (24 months) not in training, fed good quality hay with 35% concentrate as proposed by NRC, TDMI differences are erratic ± 6% between NRC and INRA systems according to the growth rate (+ 6% for INRA ration when 0.200 kg/d and - 6% when 0.450 kg/d). But the CP provided by a balance ration calculated in the INRA system are lower (- 8 to - 17%) than CP NRC requirements namely for rapid growth (- 17%). And MADC provided by a balance ration calculated in the NRC system are + 37% higher for rapid growth and + 69% for moderate growth.

Interpretation of the discrepancies are confusing by the relative NRC/INRA requirements; NRC requirements are lower than INRA requirements (table 11), and then the evolution with age and according to the growth level as well. In addition there is a strong interaction with hay-concentrate

Table 16. Comparison of rations calculated in each NRC and INRA sytems balanced for energy and protein for the growing horse.

	Yearling 12 months, Rapid growth 0.750 kg/d, BW = 320 kg					
		DM (kg)	C (%)	DE (Mcal)	CP (g)	NE (Mcal)
NRC	Hay (good)	2.80		6.55	286	3.75
	Barley	3.54		12.6	414	9.03
	Soyabean	0.66	60	2.77	359	1.58
NRC Requirements 21.7 Mcal DE 1083 g CP 2.0 < TDMI % BW <3.0	(2.2% BW)	7.00		21.92	1059	14.36
		g MADC provided by NRC ration / g MADC requirements INRA				= + 203 g MADC (+ 35%)
		DM (kg)	C (%)	NE (Mcal)	MADC (g)	DE (Mcal)
INRA	Hay (good)	2.39		3.20	120	5.59
	Barley	3.12		7.96	287	11.10
	Soyabean	0.39	60	0.93	193	1.64
INRA requirements 12.1 Mcal NE 590 g MADC 1.7 <TDMI % BW<2.5	(1.8% BW)	5.90		12.82	600	18.33
		g CP provided by INRAtion / g CP requirements NRC				= - 261 g CP (- 24%)

substitution either on DM and (or) on Nitrogen hay/concentrate ratios bases as TDMI % BW suggested by NRC (1989) are rather high and very close or (and) over to the maximum feed intake capacity of the growing horse fed hay ad libitum supplemented with very high percentage of concentrate.

Forage-concentrate substitution on DM basis is well known in growing horse in the INRA system (figure 8). Forage intake decreases in the yearling (12 months) when the amount of concentrate arises in the diet. The decreasing of the amount of forage DM intake so called substitution rate is on average 1.26 with hay (whose MADC is: 40 to 50 g MADC/kg DM) but it reaches only 0.73 for with maize silage (whose MADC is: 30 to 33 g MADC/kgDM). And the effect of substitution might rise with the age of the growing horse (Martin-Rosset and Doreau, 1984b). As a result it comes easier to understand, NRC assuming a high percentage TDMI/BW: example 2.0 - 3.0% BW for yearling (higher on average than INRA TDMI/BW: 1.7 - 2.5%, that CP requirement can be easily reach with high percentage of concentrate, even thought amount of forage intake is restricted by substitution. Conversely amount of hay intake in the INRA ration is more restricted for the substitution ratio on nitrogen basis (and energy basis as well) should be much higher due to MADC/NE ratio of hay and soyabean meal namely (tables 15-16). The figure could be discussed for the two years old as well.

In the older growing horse 2 or 3 years old, as requirement decrease intake capacity increase and ingestibility of forage are not very limiting. As a result high proportion of concentrate suggested by NRC (35%) is not appropriate in the INRA system.

For ***working horse*** direct comparisons are impossible as definition of the work intensities are different between NRC and INRA. As a result requirements are different (table 11)
After attempting adjustements of INRA work intensities and requirements to NRC proposition, comparison were attempted with good hay based diets supplemented with percentage of concentrate proposed by NRC. TDMI are higher with NRC ration than with INRA whatever the

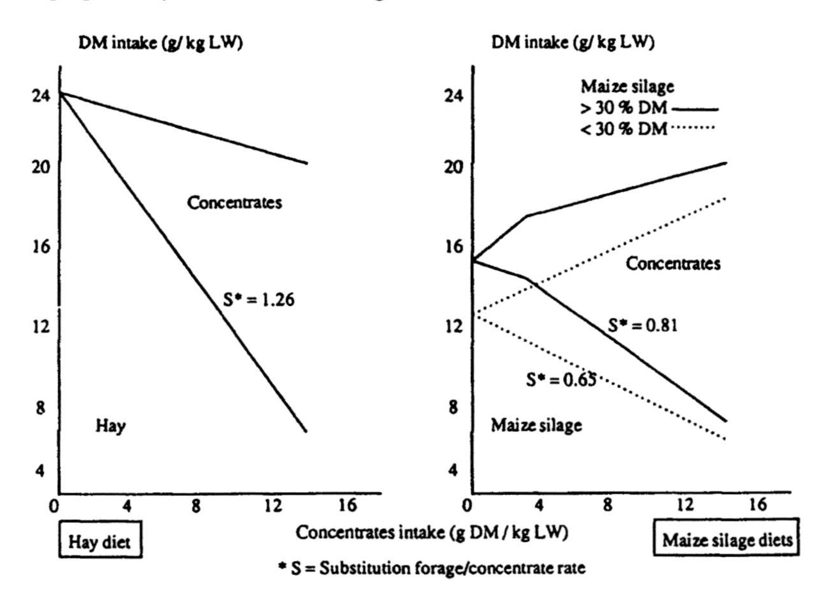

Figure 8. Effect of concentrate supplementation on forage and diet intake in young horses: 12 months of age (adapted from Agabriel et al., 1982, Martin-Rosset and Doreau 1984b).

intensities of work, but it was impossible to balance accurately INRA rations for MADC requirements - as NRC percentage of concentrate are far too high to be consistent in the INRA system. CP provided by the INRA rations were - 20 to - 27% lower than CP NRC requirements for moderate or high intensities respectively. And MADC provided by NRC rations were + 47 to + 52% higher than MADC INRA requirements for the same work intensities.

The rations were recalculated in each system with a good hay diet supplemented with lower percentage of concentrate and addition of some wheat straw to fit the MADC requirements in the INRA ration. TDMI were 2 to 19% higher for INRA rations than for NRC rations.

5.1.4 Validity of the systems

Agreement or differences in feed allowances among systems, even with the same feeds and diets do not allow conclusions to be drawn about the validity and accuracy of each system. Animal respond to inadequate rations through changes in production (milk - weight gain - exercise) body weight and body composition.
In France the validity of the MADC system was evaluated using two data files:

- Feeding trials performed at INRA with different diets based on hay, maize silage, hay-straw and supplemented with concentrates containing cereals; soyabean meal, dehy-alfalfa, bran namely, according to type of animals (growing or exercising horses). (Agabriel et al., 1982; Agabriel et al., 1984; Vermorel et al., 1984; Martin-Rosset and Doreau, 1984b; Bigot et al., 1987; Trillaud-Geyl et al., 1992; Martin-Rosset et al., 1989; Martin Rosset and Vermorel, 1991; Micol and Martin-Rosset, 1995)
- Digestion trials performed by INRA with fistulated horses for different hays or concentrates (ingredients). (Macheboeuf et al., 1995, 1996 and Martin-Rosset in progress)

5.2 Quality of protein

5.2.1 Adult

In the adult exercising horse, there is no specific nitrogen requirements (e.g. AA) clearly stated by the time when the diet provides enough energy to meet the requirements. Supplementation with branched AA (L-alnine, L-leucine, isoleucine, L-valine) provide no evidence of benefit (Casini et al., 2000; Stefanon et al., 2000). The positive effect mentioned by Glade et al. (1989) is questionable as the work bout were so mild and lactate concentration was below the anaerobic threshold. For horse at rest it has been demonstrated a long time ago (Hintz et al., 1969; Slade and Robinson, 1969...) that there is no specific AA requirements and different nitrogen source can be supplemented such as protein source: cakes or urea as well.

5.2.2 Growing horse

For the ***nursing foal***: Utilisation of milk product blend (dehyskimmed milk is preferred (Hintz et al., 1971; Borton et al., 1973) or concentrate with dehy-lactoserum (Martin-Rosset unpublished) An average of 258 and 298 g protein /kg ADG would be required at one and two months of age respectively (Doreau et al., 1986).

For the weanling soyabean meal is the best protein source as it is well balanced in indispensable AA (table 17). Other sources such as oil meals of peanut, sunflower, linseed and cotton or legumes seeds: pea, lupin, faba bean suplemented with lysine, probably as pointed out for linseed meal (which have the same lysine content as the other N source) by Hintz et al. (1971) and Wirth et al. (1973).

Table17. Amino acid content (% DM) of some feedstuffs (from table INRA 1989).

	Lysine	Threonine	Tryptophan	Methonine
Forages and by products				
dehydrated alfafa (20% CP)	1.04	0.99	0.40	0.34
alfalfa proteic concentrate	3.42	2.62	1.02	0.92
forage protein	2.69	2.71	0.44	1.08
Grains				
barley	0.43	0.40	0.13	0.20
corn	0.29	0.37	0.07	0.22
oat	0.47	0.40	0.14	0.22
Grains by products				
coarse wheat bran	0.63	0.61	0.28	0.23
corn gluten feed	0.77	0.92	0.18	0.43
Seeds				
pea (spring variety)	1.86	1.01	0.23	0.29
white soft lupin	1.93	1.48	0.32	0.32
faba bean	1.90	1.07	0.25	0.24
Cakes				
soja bean meal 50	3.47	2.14	0.74	0.75
peanut meal 50	1.87	1.46	0.54	0.54
sunflower meal	1.19	1.18	0.42	0.81
Dehydrated milk by products				
dehydrated lactic protein	7.39	4.42	1.53	2.52
dehydrated skimmed milk	2.98	1.61	0.46	0.89
skimmed lactoserum mix	1.18	0.76	0.16	0.23

The young horse expected or not to be early exercised is sensitive to quality of protein. Lysine and threonine are the first limiting amino acids. ***Yearling and 2 year old*** would require daily 33 g and 35 g of lysine respectively (e.g. 0.5% DM) or 30 g of threonine (0.4% DM) according to NRC recommandations (NRC, 1989) for lysine and preliminary data obtained by Ott et al. (1979) and Graham et al. (1994) for threonine.

For the ***non exercising long yearling or two year old*** most of N sources can be used as the AA requirements decrease and TDMI namely forage increase. Brewer dried grain could be included as well in concentrate if they are enriched with lysine (Ott et al., 1979).

6. Conclusion

In the adult, the nitrogen requirements should be refined in the future for several reasons. Nitrogen expenditures are known by everybody to be increased as far as the exercise rises but similarly nitrogen retention seems to elevate as far nitrogen intake rises too. Elevation of nitrogen expenditure provided by sustainable development of muscular mass has to be determined in relation with variation in lipids contents and their connecteced requirements. In both case knowledge of the nitrogen metabolism due to body protein turnover and synthesis and the utilization of AA as an energetic fuel througth oxydative catabolism should be improved to refine the expenditures ratio N/E which is that stated for maintenance at present.

In the young horse which have to achieve its growth and develop its muscular mass at the expense of adipose tissues, namely the long yearling and two year old, optimal tissue composition has to be determined and muscular fiber too and linked nitrogen expenditure as well.

Amount of synthetised protein are known to be related with the daily body gain, then to quantitative and qualitative nitrogen intake and ultimately at the end to energy intake as well, those last two ones having an additive effect. Simultaneously nitrogen retention elevates when nitrogen intake rises. In such a situation what are the optimal N/E and their variations in the yearling, 2 and 3 years old horse ? And finally indispensable AA out of lysine and threonine will be to be determined too.

Provided the uncertainity of the knowledge in nitrogen metabolism, the nitrogen requirements of the performances horse have to be stated with the global method: e.g. long term feeding trials for this method used to take in account for most of sources of variation. In addition the global method is in all case required to validate the requirements determined with the factorial method and to include all the environnemental effects for performing nitrogen recommanded allowances. For such a goal an appropriate nitrogen system for evaluating and expressing nitrogen value of feedstuff is requested.

The MADC system is the one which is designed at present for such a purpose. Nitrogen value is expressed as the amount of AA which are absorbed and available to cover the requirements of the host animal. The last data obtained at INRA in the year nineties supported the amount of protein digested in the small intestine. Then ideal protein for the different kind of horses have to be determined.

From the work done by different workers, it is known that there is no AA absorption in the large intestine. As a result the next challenge to refine the MADC system should be the determination of N requirements of the microflora in the large intestine, whose role is to provide energy to host animal. It is likely that the N microflora requirement might be close to AA recovery rate stated by INRA in 1984-1994 (10 to 30% of alimentary protein digested in the large intestine) where there was still an incertainity about AA absorption in the large intestine.

Referring to present knowledge, the MADC system allows to express with an acceptable accuracy the amount of AA which are required to cover the requirements of host animal and those of microflora in the large intestine. And those recommandations have been tested in the different situation through long term feeding trials.

References

Agabriel, J., Trillaud-Geyl, C., Martin-Rosset, W. and Jussiaux, M., 1982. Utilisation de l'ensilage de maïs par le poulain de boucherie. INRA Prod. Anim., 49: 5-13.

Apparent digestion in various segments of the digestive tract of ponies fed diets with varying roughage-grain ratio. J. Anim. Sci., 32: 10-102.

Agabriel, J., Martin-Rosset, W. and Robelin, J., 1984. Croissance et besoins du populain. Chapitre 22. In: R. Jarrige, W. Martin-Rosset Editor « Le cheval » INRA publications, route de St Cyr, 78000 Versailles. 370-384.

Almeida, F.Q., Valdares, Filho, S.C., Donzelz, J.L., Coelho Da Silva, J.F., Queiroz, A.C. and Cecon, P.R., 1999. Prececal digestibility of aminoacids in diets for horses. In 16th Eq. Nutr. Phys. Symp. North Raleigh Carolina US. p. 274-279.

Austbo, D., 1996. Energy and protein evaluation systems and nutritent recommendations for horses in the nordic countries. In: Proceedings of the 47th European Asscoaitions of Animal Production Meeting. Lillehammer, Norway, august 26-29, abstract H4.4, p. 293. Wageningen Pers. Ed. Wageningen, The Netherlands.

Baruc, C.I., Dawson, K.A. and Baker, I.P., 1983. -The characherization and nitrogen metabolism of equine caecal bacteria. 8th ENPS, Kentucky, April, 28-30, p. 151-156..

Bertone, A.L., Van Soest, P.I. and Stashak, T.D., 1989. Digestion, fecal and b1ood variables associated with extensive large colon resection in the horse. Am. I. Vel. Res., 50: 253-258.

Bigot, G., Trillaud-Geyl, C., Jussiaux, M. and Martin-Roset, W., 1987. Elevage du cheval de selle du sevrage au débourrage: alimentation hivernale, croissance et développement. INRA Prod. Anim. 69: 45-53.

Bochroder, B., Schubert, R. Bodecker, D. and Holler, M., 1992. In vitro transit of basic amino acids in the ventral colon of the horse. In kongressband 1992, Gottingen.

Bochroder, B., Schubert, R. and Bodecker, D., 1994. Studies on the transport in vitro of lysine, histidine, arginine and ammonia across the mucosa of the equine colon. Equine Veterinary journal, 26 (2) 131-133.

Booth, F.W. and Watson, P.A., 1985. Control of adaptations in protein levels in reponse to exercise. Fed. Proc. 44: 2292.

Borton, A., Anderson, D.L. and Lyford, S., 1973. Studies of protein quality and quantity in the early weaned foal. Proc. 3rd Equine Nutrition and Physiology Symposium. University of Florida, Gainesville, 19-22.

Breuer, L.H., Kasten, K.H. and Word, J.D., 1970. Protein and amino acid utilization in the young horse. In: Proc. 2nd Equine Nutrition Research Symposium. Cornel University, Ithaca, 16-17.

Breuer, L.H. and Gloden, D.L., 1971. Lysine requirements of the immature equine. J. Anim. Sci., 33: 227.

Cabrera, L. and Tisserand, J.L., 1995. Effet du rythme de distribution et de la fonne de distribution d'un régime paille concentrée sur l'aminoacidémie chez le poney. Ann. Zootech., 44: 105-114.

Casini, L., Gatta, D., Magni, L. and Colombani, B., 2000. Effect of prolonged branched-chain amino acid supplementation on metabolic response to anaerobic exercise in Standardbreds. J. Equuine Vet. Sci., 20: 120-123.

Coleman, R.J., Mathison, G.W., Hardin, R.T. and Milligan, J.P., 2001. Effect fo dietary forge and protein concentration on total tract, prececal and post ileal protein and lysine digestibilities of forage based-diets fed to mature ponies. In 17th Eq. Nut. Phys. Symp. Lexington KY May 31 - June 2nd USA. p. 461-463.

Cordelet, C., 1990. Contribution à l'étude de l'alimentation azoté du cheval: utilisation de la fraction azotée dans le gros intestin. Mémoire Ingénieur CNAM. Dijon. 94 pp.

Crandell, K., Pagan, J.D., Harris, P. and Duren, S.E., 2001. A comparison of grain, vegetable oil and beet pulp as energy sources for the exercised horse. In advances in Equine Nutrition II, KER Ed. Lexington KY USA p. 487.

Cuddeford, D., 1997. Feeding systems for horses. Chap. 11. In: Feeding systems and feed evaluation models. Theodorou, M.K. France J., Ed. Cabi Publishing, Oxon, UK, NY, USA, p. 239-274.

Doreau, M., Boulot, S., Martin-Rosset, W. and Robelin, J., 1986. Relation between nutrient intake, growth and body composition of nursing foal. Reprod. Nutr. Develop., 26 (2B): 683-690.

Eckersall, P.D., Kerr, M.G. and Snow, D.H., 1982. Cited par Meyer, 1983.

Essen Gustavson, B., Bloomstrand, E., Karlstrom, K., 1991. Influence of diet on substrate metabolism during exercise. In Proceeding 4th ICEEP, p. 288.

Frank, N.B., Meachyam, T.N., Easley, K.J. and Fontenot, J.P., 1983. The effect of by-passing the small intestine on nutrient digestibility and absorption in the pony. In 8th Eq. Nutr. Phys. Symp. Lexington KY. USAp. 243-248.

Frape, D., 1998. Equine nutrition and feeding. 2nd Ed. Blackwell. Science Ltd, London, pp. 564.

Freeman, D.W., Potter, G.D., Schelling, G.T. and Kreider, J.L., 1985a. Nitrogen metabolism in the mature physically conditionned horse. I. Response to donctiioning. 9th Eq. Nut. Phys. Symp. Michigan University, 230-235.

Freeman, D.W., Potter, G.D., Schelling, G.T. and Kreider, J.L., 1985b. Nitrogen metabolism in the mature physically conditionned horse. II. Response to varying nitrogen intake. 9th Eq. Nut. Phys. Symp. Michigan University. 236-241.

Friedman, J.E. and Lemon, P.W.R., 1989. Effect of chronic endurance exercise on retention of dietary protein. Int. J. Sports Med. 10(2), 118.

Gibbs, F.G., Fotter, G.D., Schelling, G.T. and Kremer I-L. Boyd, C.L., 1988. Digestion of hay protein in differents segments of the equine digestive tract. J. Anim., 66: 400-406.

Gibbs, F.G., Potter, G.D., Schilling, G.T., Kreider, J.L., Boyd, C.L., 1996. The significance of small vs large intestine digestion of cereal grain and oil seed protein in the equine. J. Equine Vet. Sci., 162, 60.

Glade, M.J., 1983. Nitrogen partitioning along the equine digestive tract. I. Anim. Sci., 57: 943-953.

Glade, M.J., 1984, The influence of dietary fiber digestibility on the nitrogen requirements of mature horses. I. Anim. Sci., 58: 638-646.

Glade, M.J., 1989. Effects of specific amino acid supplementtion on lactic acid production by horses exercised on a treadmill. Proc. Eleventh Equine Nutr. Physiol. Symp., 244.

Godbee, R.G. and Slade, L.M., 1979. Nitrogen absorption from the cecum of a mature horse. In;Froc. 6th Equine Nutrition and Physiology Symposium. Texas A.M. University, 75-76.

Graham, P.M., Ott, E.A., Brendemuhl, J.H. and Tenbroeck, S.H., 1994. The effect of supplemental lysine and threonine on growth and development of yearling horses. J. Anim. Sci., 72: 380-386.

Graham-Thiers, P.M., Kronfeld, D.S., Kline, K.A., Mc Cullough, T.M. and Harris, P.A., 1999. Dietary protein level and proetin status during exercise, training and stall rst. 16th Equine Nutr. Phys. Sym. Raleigh, NC, p. 104-105.

Hintz, F., Lowe, J.E. and Schryver, H.F., 1969. Protein sources for horses. Proc. Cornelle Nutr..Conf. 65-68.

Hintz, H.F., Rogue, D.E., WAlker, E.F., Lowe, I.E. and Schryver, H.F., 1970. Apparent digestion in various segments of the digestive tract of ponies fed diets with varying roughage-grain ratio. J. Anim. Sci., 32: 10-102.

Hintz, H.F., Schryver, H.F. and Lowe, J.E., 1971. Comparison of a blend of milk products and linseedmeal as protein supplements for young growing horses. J. Anim. Sci., 33: 1274-1277.

Hintz, H.F., Schryver, H.F., 1972. Nitrogen utilization in ponies. J. Anim. Sci., 34: 592-595.

Hintz, H.F., White, K.K., Short, C.E., Lowe, J.E. and Ross, M., 1980. Effects of protein levels on endurance horses. J. Anim. Sci. 51: Sup. 202-203.

Hintz, H.F. and Cymbaluck, N.F., 1994. Nutrition of the horse. Ann. Rev. 14: 243-267.

Houpt, T.R. and Houpt, K., 1971. Nitrogen conservation by ponies fed a low-protein ration Am. J. Vet. Res., 32: 579-588.

INRA, 1984. Tables de la valeur nutritive des aliments pour le cheval. In: R. Jarrige, W. Martin-Rosset Editors. « Le Cheval » Reproduction, Sélection, Alimentation, Exploitation. R. Jarrige et W. Martin-Rosset Editors. INRA Editions Route de St Cyr, 78000 Versailles pp. 661-689.

INRA, 1984. Tables des apports alimentaires recommandés 643-660 et tables de la valeur nutritive des aliments pour le cheval. 661-689. ln: Jarrige R., Martin-Rosset W. (Editors). "Le Cheval" Reproduction -Sélection -Alimentation -Exploitation. INRA Publications, Route de St Cyr, 78000 Versailles.

INRA, 1984. Le Cheval: Reproduction, Sélection, Alimentation, Exploitatio. R. Jarrige et W. Martin-Rosset Editors. INRA Editions Route de St Cyr, 78000 Versailles pp. 689.

INRA, 1984. Tables des apports alimentaires recommandés pour le cheval. In: R. Jarrige, W. Martin-Rosset Editors. « Le Cheval » Reproduction, Sélection, Alimentation, Exploitation. R. Jarrige et W. Martin-Rosset Editors. INRA Editions Route de St Cyr, 78000 Versailles pp. 645-660.

INRA, 1988. Ruminant Nutrition. R. Jarrige Ed., INRA Editions, Route de St-Cyr, 78026 Versailles, pp. 389.

INRA, 1990. L'alimentation des chevaux. W. Martin-Rosset Editors. « Le cheval » INRA Editions Route de St Cyr, 78000 Versailles pp. 232.

INRA, 1978. Alimentation des ruminants Jarrige R. (Ed). INRA Publications, Route de St Cyr, 78000 Versailles, 597 pp.

Jarrige, R. and Tisserand, J.L., 1984. Métabolisme, besoins et alimentation azotée du cheval. Chapter 18. In: R. Jarrige, W. Martin-Rosset Editors. « Le Cheval » Reproduction, Sélection, Alimentation, Exploitation. R. Jarrige et W. Martin-Rosset Editors. INRA Editions Route de St Cyr, 78000 Versailles pp. 277-302.

Jordan, R.M. and Myers, V., 1972. Effect of protein levels on the growth of wean eanling and yearling ponies. J. Anim. Sci., 34: 578-581.

Julliand, V. and Tisserand, J.L., 1992. Alimentation du poeny: importance de la qualité de l'azote sur la flore microbienne caecale. In 18e J. Rech. Eq. Paris 4 mars p. 1-11.

Julliand, V., 1998. Ecologie microbienne du système digestif des équidés. Nouvelles approches, conséquences. In Proceeding 24e Journée Recherche Equine, Paris, 4 Mars, 105-114.

Kellner, O., 1879. Untersuchungen uber den zysammenhang zwischen muskelthatigkeit und stoffzerfall im thierischen organismus. Landwirtschaftschaflishe Jahrbücher, 8: 701-712.

Kellner, O.,1880. Untersuchungen uber den zysammenhang zwischen muskelthatigkeit und stoffzerfall im thierischen organismus. Landwirtschaftschaflishe Jahrbücher, 9: 651-688.

Kellner, O., 1909. Principes fondamentaux de l'alimentation du bétail. 3me Ed. Allemande,Traduction A Gregoire Berger Levault, Paris, Nancy, 288 pp.

Lawrence W., 1998. Protein requirements of equine athltetes. In K. Pagan Editor. Advances in Equine Nutrition. Nottingham Univ. Press. Ed. p. 161-166.

Lemon, P.W.R., 1991. Proctor DN Protein intake and athletic performance. Sports Med. 12(5): 313.

Lemon, P.W.R., Tarnopolsky, M.A., Macdouglall, J.D. et al., 1992. Protein requirements and muscle mass/strength changes during intesnive training in novice bodybuilders. J. Appl. Physiol. 73(2), 767.

Lindsay, D.B., 1980. Amino acids as energy sources. Proc. Nutr. Soc., 39: 53-59.

Lindsay, D.B., 1982. Relationship between amino acid catabolism and protein anabolism in the ruminants. Federatin Proc., 41, 2550-2554.

Lucke, J.N. and Hall, G.M., 1980. Long distance exercise in the horse: golden Horseshoe Ride 1978. Veterinary Record, 106: 405-407.

Macheboeuf, D., Marangi, M., Poncet, C. and Martin-Rosset, W., 1995. Study of nitrogen digestion from different hays by the mobile nylon bag technique in horses. Ann. Zootech., 44, suppl. 219 (abstract).

Macheboeuf, D., Poncet, C., Jestin, M. and Martin-Rosset, C., 1996. Use of a mobile nylon bag technique with caecum fistulated horses as an alternative method for estimating pre-caecal and total tract nitrogen digestibilities of feedstuffs. In: Proceedings fo the 47th European Association of Animal Production Meeting. Lillehammer, Norway, august 26-29, Abstract H4.9, p. 296. Wageningen The Netherlands.

Maczuluck, A.E., Dawson, K.A. and Baker, J.P., 1983. In vitro nitrogen utilization by equine caecal bacterial. In 8th Eq. Nut. Phys. Symp. Lexington KY. USA p. 255-258.

Martin-Rosset, W., Boccard, R., Jussiaux, M., Robelin, J. and Trillaud-Geyl, 1983b. Croissance relative des différents tissus, organes et régions corporelles entre 12 et 30 mois chez le cheval de boucherie de différentes races lourdes. Ann. Zootech. 32: 153-174.

Martin-Rosset, W., Andrieu, J., Vermorel, M. and Dulphy, J.P., 1984a. Valeur nutritive des aliments pour le cheval. Chapter 17. In: R. Jarrige, W. Martin-Rosset Editors. « Le Cheval » INRA Editions Route de St Cyr, 78000 Versailles p. 208-239.

Martin-Rosset, W. and Doreau, M., 1984b. Consommation des aliments et d'eau par le cheval. Chapter 22. In Jarrige R., Martin-Rosset W. Editor « Le cheval » INRA Editin Route de St-Cyr 78000 Versailles, p. 334-354.

Martin-Rosset, W. and Dulphy, J.P., 1987. Digestibility. Interactions between forages and concentrates in horses: influence of feeding level. Comparison with sheep. Livest. Prod. Sci., 17: 263-276.

Martin-Rosset, W., Tavernier, L. and Vermorel, M., 1989. Alimentation du cheval de club avec un régime à base de paille et d'aliments composés. Proceedings 15e Journée Recherche Chevaline. Paris 8 mars. CEREOPA Ed. 16 rue Claude Bernard 75231 Paris Cedex 05, p. 90-102.

Martin-Rosset, W., Vermorel, M., Doreau, M., Tisserand, J.L. and Andrieu, J., 1994. The french horse feed evaluation systems and recomended allowances for energy and protein. Livest. Prod. Sci. 40: 37-56.

Martin-Rosset, W., Vermorel, M., Doreau, M., Tisserand, J.L. and Andrieu, J., 1994. The french horse feed evaluation systems and recommended allowances for energy and protein. -,Livest. Prod. Sci., 40: 37 -56.

Martin-Rosset, W., 2001. Croissance osseuse chez le cheval In 27th J. Rech. Eq. Paris 7 mars. 73-100.

Mc Ilwraith, C.W., 2001. Developmental orthopaedic diseases (DOD) in horses. A multifactorial process. In 17th Eq. Nutr. Phys. Symp. Lexington KY. USA 1-23.
Mc Meniman, N.P., Elliot, R., Groenendyk, S. and Dowsetf, K.F., 1987. Synthesis and absorption of cysteine from the hindgut of the horse. Equine vet. J. 19: 192-194.
Meakin, D.W. and Hintz, H.F., 1984. The effect of dietary protein on calcium metabolism and growth of the weanling foal. Proc. Cornell Nutr. Conf. 95-102.
Meyer, H. and Peerdekamp, M., 1980. Auswirkungen überhöhter proteingaben beim pferd. Azbl. Vet. Med., A27: 756-757.
Meyer, H., 1983. Protein metabolism and protein requirements in horses. In: IVème Symposium International Métabolisme et Nutrition Azotés. Clennont-Ferrand. Arnal M.. Pion R., Bonind., (Editors). Vol 1: 343-374. Les colloques de l'INRA, na 16, INRA publications, Route de St Cyr,78000 Versailles.
Meyer, H., 1987. Nutrition of the equine athlete. In: Proceedings 2nd Equine exercise Physiology Symposium, Gillepsie J.P., Robinson N.E., Editors. ILEEP Publications. Davis, USA, p. 644.
Meyer, H., Radiche, S., Kienzle, E., Wilke, S. and Keffken, D., 1993 -Investigations on preileal digestion of oats, corn and barley starch in relation to grain processing. Proc. 13th ENPS, Florida, January 21-23: 92-97.
Meyer, H., Radicke, S., Kienzle, H., Wilke, S. and Kleffen, D., 1993. Investigations on preileal digestion of oat, corn and barley starch in relation to grain processing. In: Proceedings 13th Equine Nutrition and Physiology Symoposium, January 21-23. Gainsesville.Florida, USA. p. 66-71.
Micol, D., Martin-Rosset, W., 1995. Feeding systems for horses on high forage diet in the temperate zone. In Proceeding Clermont-Fd, sept. 11-15th, INRA Editions, Versailles, 569-584
Miller, P.A. and Lawrence, L.M., 1988. The effect of dietary protein level on exercising horses. J. Anim. Sci. 66: 2185.
Miller-Graber, P.A., Lawrence, L.M., Foreman, J.H. et al., 1991a. Dietary protein level and energy metabolism during treadmill exercise in horses. J. Nutr. 121: 1462.
Miller-Graber, P.A., Lawrence, L.M., Foreman, J.H. et al., 1991b. Effect of dietary protein level on nitrogen metabolites in exercised Quater Horses. Equine Exer. Physiol., 3: 305.
Miller-Graber, P.A., Lawrence, L.M., Kurcz, E., Kane, R., Bump, K., Fisher, M. and Smith, J., 1990. The free amino acid profile in the middle gluteal before and after fatiguing exercise in the horse. Equine Vet. J., 22: 209-210.
Millward, D.J., Davies, C.T., Halliday, D., Wolman, S.L., Matthews, D. and Rennie, M., 1982. Effect of exercise on protein metabolism in humans explored with stable isotopes. Federation Proc., 41: 2686-2691.
Millward, D.J., Bates, P.C., De Benoist, B., Brown, J.G., Cox, M., Halliday, D., Odedra, B. and Rennie, M.J., 1983. Protein turnover. The nature of the phenomena and its physiological regualtion. In: Ive Symposium Int. Métabolisme et Nutrition azotés. Clermont-Ferrand (Ed. M. Aranl, R. Pion et D. Bonin) Vol. 1, 69-96. Les colloques de l'INRA, n° 16. INRA Publications. Route de Saint-Cyr, 78000 Versailles.
Miraglia, N. and Oliveri, O., 1990. Statement and expression of the energy and nitrogen value of feedstuffs in Southern Europe. In: Proceedings of the 41st European Association of Animal Production Meeting. Toulouse, France, Abstract p. 390. Wageningen Pers. Ed. The Netherlands.
Moore-Colyer, M.J.S., Longland, A.C., Hyslop, J.J. and Cuddeford, D., 1998. The degradation of protein and non-starch polysaccharides (NSP) from botanically diverse sources of dietary fiber by ponies as measured by the mobile bag technique. In: In vitro Techbniques for Measuring Nutrients Supply to Ruminants. Occasional Publication n° 22, BSAS, Penicuik, Edinburgh.
National Research Council, 1989. Nutrients requirements of domestic animals, n° 6. Nutrients Requirements of Horses. 5th Revised Edition. National Academy of Sciences, Washington, D.C. pp. 100.
Nicoletti, J.N., Wohlt, J. and Glade, M.J., 1980. Nutrition utilization by ponies and steers as affected by dietary forage rations. J. Anim. Sci. 51, supl. 1: 25.
NRC, 1978 -National Research Councel, Nutriment requirements of horses. 4th revised edition Ed National Academy of Sciences, Washington USA, vol 6: 1-33.
Oldham, J.D. and Lidsay, D.B., 1983. Interraltionships between protein-yielding and energy-yielding nutrients. In: Ive Sympsoium Int. Metaboisme et Nutrition azotés. Clermont-Ferrand (Ed. M. Aranl, R. Pion et D. Bonin) Vol. 1, 183-209. Les colloques de l'INRA, n° 16. INRA Publications. Route de Saint-Cyr, 78000 Versailles.

Olsson, N. and Ruudvere, A., 1955. The nutrition of the horse. Nutr. Abs. Rev., 25: 1-18.
Ott, E.A., Asquith, R.L., Feaster, J.P. and Martin, F.G., 1979. Influence of protein level and quality on the growth and development of yearling foals. J. Anim., Sci., 49: 620-628.
Ott, E.A., Asquith, R.L. and Feaster, J.P., 1981. Lysine supplementation of diets for yearling horses. J. Anim. Sci., 53: 1496-1503.
Ott, E.A., Asquith, R.L., 1983. Influence of protein and mineral intake on growth and bone development of weanling horses. In Proceeding, 8th ENPS, Lexington, Kentucky, USA, April 28-30th: 39-44.
Ott, E.D., 2001. Protein and aminoacids. In Advances in Equine Nutrition J.D. Pagan and R.J. Geor Ed. Nottingham Universitu Press. Nottingham. UK 237-246.
Pagan, J.D., Essen-Gustavsson, B., Lindohlm, M. and Thornton, J., 1987. The effect of dietary energy source on exercise performance in Standard-bred horses. In: Proceediings, 2nd Exercise Physiology Symposium, Gillepsie J.R. Robinson N.E., Editions ICEEP Publications, Davis, USA, p. 686-701.
Patterson, P.H., Coon, C.N. and Hughes, J.M., 1985. Protein requirements of mature workin horses. J. Anim. Sc. 61: 187.
Potter, G.D., Gibbs, P.G., Haley, R.G. and Klendshoj, C., 1992. Digestion of protein in the small and large intestines of Equine fed mixed diets. Proc. Europaïsche Konferenz über die Ernahrung des Pferdes. 3-4 september Hannover. pp. 140-143.
Potter, G.D., Gibbs, P.G., Haley, R.G. and Klendshoj, C., 1992b. Digestion of protein in the small and large intestine of equines fed mixed diets. In: Proceedings 1st European Conference on Horse Nutrition, Hannover, Geramny, pp. 140-143.
Prior, R.L., Hintz, H.F., Lowe, J.E. and Visek, W.J., 1974. Urea recycling and metabolism of ponies. J. Anim. Sci., 38: 565-571.
Reeds, P.J., Fukller M.F., 1983. Nutrient intake and protein turnover. Proc. Nutr. Soc. 42: 463-471.
Reeds P.J. and Harris, C.I., 1981. Protein turnover in animals: man in his context. In: Nitrogen metabolism in Man (Ed. J.C. Waterlow et J.M.L. Stephen). Applied Science Pub., London. 391-402.
Reitnour, C.M., Baker, J-P., Mitchel, G.E. Jr and Little, C.O., 1969. Nitrogen digestion in different segments of the equine digestive tract. J. Anim. Sci., 29: 332-334.
Reitnour, C.M. and Salsbury, R.L., 1976. Utilization of proteins by the equine species. Am. J. Vet. Res., 37:1065-1067.
Reitnour, C.M., 1979. Effect of caecal administrtion of corn starch on nitrogen metabolism in ponies. J. Anim. Sci. 49: 988-992.
Reitnour, C.M., 1980. Protein utilization in response to caecal corn starch in ponies. J. Anim. Sci. 51, Sup. 1: 218.
Rennie, M.J., Edwards, R.T.H., Halliday, D., Davies, C.T.M., Matthews, D.E. and Millward, D.J., 1981. Protein metabolism during exercise. In: Nitrogen metabolism in Man (Ed. J.C. Waterlow et J.M.L. Stephen). Applied Science Pub., London. 509.
Rerat, A., 1981. Contribution du gros intestin à la digestion des glucides et des matièers azotées chez le monogastrique omnivore. Reprod. Nutr. Dévelop., 21 (5B): 815-847.
Robinson, D.W. and Slade, L.M., 1974. The current status of knowledge on the nutrition of Equines. J. Anim. Sci., 39: 1045-1066.
Rogers, P., Albert, W.W. and Fahey, G.C., 1981. Blood aminoacid profiles of gestating and lactating mares fed diets with and without lysine and methionine. In: Proc. 7th Equine nutrition and physiology Symposium. Warenton. Virginia, 73-78.
Saastamoinen, M.T. and Kosiknen, E., 1993. Influence of quality of dietary protein supplement and anabolic steroids on muscular and sleletal growth of foals. Anim. Prod; 56 (1): 135-144.
Satabin, P., Bois-Joyeux, B., Chanez, M. et al., 1989a. Effects of long-term feeding of high-protein or high-fat diets on the response to exercise iin the rat. Eur. Appl. Physiol. 58: 583.
Satabin, P., Bois-Joyeux, B., Chanez, M. et al., 1989b. Post-exercise glycogen resynthesis in trained high-protein or high -fat-fed rats after glucose feeding. Eur. Appl. Physiol., 58: 591.
Savage, C.J., Mc Carthy, R.N. and Jeffcott, L.B., 1993. Effect of dietary energy and protein on induction of dyschondroplasia in foals. Equine Vet. J., 16: 74-79.

Schmidt, M., Lindemann, G. and Meyer, H., 1982. Intestinaler N-umsatz beim Pferd. Adv. Anim. Physiol. And Anim. Nutr. 13: 40-51 Parey Hamburg.

Schmitz, M., Abrens, F. and Hagemeister, H., 1990 -Beitrag der Absorption von Aminosauren im Dikdarrn zur Proteinversorgung bei Pferd, Rind und Schwein. J. Animal Physiol. Animal Nutr. 64: 12-13.

Slade, L.M., Robinson, D.W. and Casey, K.E., 1970. Nitrogen metabolism in non-ruminant herbivores. I. The influence of non-protein and protein quality on the nitrogen retention of adult mares. J. Anim. Sci., 30: 753-760.

Slade, L.M., Bishop, R., Morris, J.G. and Robinson, D.M., 1971. Digestion and absorption of 1SN-Iabelled microbial protein in the large intestine of the horse Br. Vet. J. 127: XI-XlII.

Slade, L.M., Robinson, D.W. and Al-Rabbat, F., 1973. Ammonia turnover in the large intestine. In 3rd Eq. Nut. Phy. Symp. Gainesville. Florida USA p. 1-12.

Slade, L.M., Lewis, D., Quinn, C. and Chandler, L., 1975. Nutritional adaptation of horses for endurance performance. In: Proc. 4th Equine nutrition and physiology Symposium. Davis, 114-128.

Slade, L.M., Robinson, D.W. and Al-Rabbat, F., 1973. Ammonia turnover in the large intestine. In Proceedings 3th Equine Nutrition Physiology Symposium, Gainesville, Florida, USA, p. 1-12.

Smolders, E.A.A., 1990. Evolution of the energy and nitrogen systems used in the Netherlands. In: Proceedings of the 41st European Association of Animal Production Meeting. Toulouse France, p. 386 (abstract). Wageningen Pers. Ed. Wageningen The Netherlands.

Snow, D.H., Kerr, M.G., Nimmo, M.A. and Abbott, E.M., 1982. Alterations in blood, sweat, urine and muscle composition during prolonged exercise in the horse. Vet. Rec., 110: 377-384.

Staun, H., 1990. Energy and nitrogen systems used in northern countries for estimating and expressing value of feedstuffs in horses. In: Proceedings of the 41st European Association of Animal Production Meeting. Toulouse France, p. 388. Wageningen Pers. Ed. Wageningen The Netherlands.

Stefanon, B., Bettini, C. and Guggia, P., 2000. Administration of branched-chain amino acids to Standardbred horses in training. J. Equine Vet. Sci., 20: 115-119.

Tisserand. J.L. and Martin-Rosset, W., 1996. Evaluation of the protein value of feedstuffs in horses in the MADC system. In Proceeding of 47th Annual Meeting of European Association for Animal Production. Lillehammer August 25-29 Norway. Aleshat H.4.3. p. 293. Wageningen Pers. Ed. Wageningen The Netherlands. (Full paper p. 13).

Trillaud-Geyl, C., Bigot, G., Jurquet, V., Bayle, M., Arnaud, G., Dubroeucq, H., Jussiaux, M. and Martin-Rosset, W., 1992. Influence du niveau de croissance pondérale sur le développement squelettique du cheval de sell. In 18e J. Rech. Eq; Paris 4 mars 162-168.

Vermorel, M., Vernet, J. and Martin-Rosset W., 1997. Digestive and energy utilization of two diets by ponies nd horses. Livest. Prod. Sci. 51: 13-19.

Willmore, J.H. and Freund Beau, J., 1984. Nutritional enhancement of athletic performance. Nutr. Abs. Rev. Series A., 54: 1-16.

Winkel, C., 1977. Untersuchungen über Schweissmenge und zusammensetzung des Pferdes unter beonderer Berücksichtigung der Eiweissversorgung. Vet. Diss. Hannover.

Wirth, B.L., Potter, G.D. and Broderick, G.A., 1973. Colton seed meal and lysine for weanling foal. In J. Anim. Sci. 37, n° 200 (abstract).

Wysocki, Aa. and Baker, J.P., 1975. Utilization of bacterial protein from the lower gut of the equine. In: Proc. 4th Equine nutrition and physiology Symposium. Ca1ifornia University. Pomona 21.

Young, V., 1986. Protein and amino acid metabolism in relation to physical exercise. In: Winnick M. (ed) Nutrition and Exercise. John Wiley and Sons, NY, 9.

The Dutch net protein system

Andrea D. Ellis

Research Institute for Animal Husbandry, Lelystad, The Netherlands

1. Protein requirements for horses

In the Dutch system protein requirements are given in apparent digestible crude protein (Digestible Crude Protein horses - VREp). Requirements have been derived from the German system (DLG, 1982) which calculates protein digestibility by multiplying feed CP with the apparent faecal digestibility coefficient. It is therefore not directly comparable with the French system, which corrects with a co-efficient for apparent pre-caecal digestibility (MADC).

The CVB uses the **3 g VREp/BW $^{0.75}$** as determined by Meyer (1992) for maintenance requirements of adult horses.

DLG, NRC and INRA keep a constant relationship between protein requirements and energy requirements. This can lead to an overestimation of protein requirements as with increasing work the energy requirements increases to a much greater extent than protein requirements. Therefore, this relationship should be seen as general advise only, in view of a general lack of knowledge as to true protein requirements.

Following the maintenance requirements for energy at 39 VEP/kg BW$^{0.75}$ for Thoroughbred and Warmblood horses (mares/geldings) and a 3g VREp requirement a relationship of 13:1 in the ration can be established. This relationship is maintained in the recommendations for working horses in the Dutch system, so the energy (VEP) increase for maintenance and work divided by 13 give the required DCP (VREp) increase (Table 5).

Table 1. Protein requirements (VREp) for maintenance and additional requirements per hour work.

Horse BW (kg)	Maintenance	Rider (kg)	Walk	Light	Medium	Heavy work	Very heavy
100	95	45	15	25	35	45	90
200	160	50	25	40	60	75	170
300	215	55	35	55	80	105	235
400	270	60	45	75	110	135	305
500	315	70	55	85	130	165	375
600	365	80	65	105	160	200	450
700	410	90	75	120	180	230	520
800	450	90	85	140	205	260	585

(Source: CVB 1996)

2. Example requirement calculations for performance horses

On the next page some examples are given of how a computer program can calculate energy and protein requirements for the performance horse. The shaded boxes need to be filled in by the horse owner. Under 'Work' average speed of paces is given, but under 'Speed m/min' these can be adapted (see Eventer). Examples are given for horses at professional level.

Maintenance	SHOWJUMPER		DRESSAGE		EVENTING	
Horse Weight	600 kg		550 kg		580 kg	
Energy and Protein	VEP	VREp	VEP	VREp	VEP	VREp
Maintenance Requirements	4728	364	4429	341	4609	355
Work	Speed m/min	Minutes	Speed m/min	Minutes	Speed m/min	Minutes
walk, 120m/min	120	20	120	50	120	45
trot, 240m/min	240	20	240	30	240	10
trot, 540m/min	540	0	540	10	540	10
galop, 360m/min	360	10	360	10	300	20
galop, 720m/min	720	0	720		360	10
jumping, 400m/min	400	20	400		400	10
Rider and Tack (kg)		80		65		70
Requirements for work	VEP	VREp	VEP	VREp	VEP	VREp
Energy and Protein	3118	240	3712	286	4901	377
Total Requirements	7846	604	8141	626	9510	732

References

Armsby, H.P., 1903. The principles of Animal Nutrition, Chapman & Hall, London.

Brody, S., 1945. Bioenergetics and Growth, Reinhold Publishing Coporation, New York.

DLG, 1992. Epfehlungen zur Energie- und Nahrstoffversorgung der Pferde, DLG-Verlag, Frankfurt/Main.

CVB, 1996. Documentatierrapport nr 15, Het definitieve VEP- en VREp-systeem, centraal veevoederbureau.

CVB, 2000. Veevoedertabel 2000, Centraal Veevoederbureau, Lelystad.

INRA, 1984. Jarrige, R. and Martin-Rosset, W. (eds.) Le Cheval, Reproduction, Selection, Alimentation, Exploitation, Instituut National de la Recherche Argronomique, Paris.

Martin-Rosset, W. and Dulphy, J.P., 1987. Digestibility Interactions between Forages and Concentrates in Horses: Influence of Feeding Level - Comparison with Sheep, Livestock Production Science, 17, 263-276.

Martin-Rosset, W., Doreau, M., Boulot, S. and Miraglia, N., 1990. Influence of level of feeding and physiological state on diet digestibility in light and heavy breed horses, Livestock Production Science, 25: 257-264.

Martin-Rosset, W. and Vermorel, M., 1991. Maintenance energy requirements determined by indirect calorimetry and feeding trials in light horses, Equine Veterinary Science, 11: 42-45.

Martin-Rosset, W., Vermorel, M., Doreau, M., Tisserand, J.L., Andrieu, J., 1994. The French Horse Feed Evaluation System and Recommended Allowances for Energy and Protein, Livestock Production Science, 40: 37-57, INRA.

Meyer, H., 1992. Pferdefütterung, 2. Auflage, Blackwell Wissenschafts-Verlag, Berlin, Wien.

NRC, 1989. Nutrient Requirements of Horses, 5th ed. revised, National Academy of Sciences, Washington DC.

Pagan, J.D. and Hintz, H.F., 1986. Equine Energetics. I: Relationship between body weight and energy requirements in horses, J. Anim. Sci., 63: 815-821.

Vermorel, M., Martin-Rosset, W. and Vernet, J., 1997a. Energy utilisation of twelve forages or mixed diets for maintenance by sport horses, Livestock Production Sciences, 47: 157-167.

Vermorel, M., Vernet, J. and Martin-Rosset, W., 1997b. Digestive and energy utilisation of two diets by ponies and horses, Livestock Production Science, 51: 13-19.

Vermorel, M. and Martin-Rosset, W., 1997. Concepts, scientific basis, structure and validation of the French horse net energy system (UFC), Livestock Production Science, 47: 261-275.

Vernet, J., Vermorel, M. and Martin-Rosset, W., 1995. Energy cost of eating long hay, straw and pelleted food in sport horses, Animal Science, 61: 581-588.

Smolders, E.A.A., 1987. Energy requirements during maximal exercise, EAAP, Lissabon.

Smolders, E.A.A., Steg, A. and Hindle, V.A., 1990. Organic Matter Digestibility in Horses and its Prediction, Netherlands Journal of Agricultural Science, 38: 435-447.

Evaluating the protein requirements of horses: The German system for digestible crude protein

M. Coenen

School of Veterinary Medicine Hannover, Department of Animal Nutrition

In comparison to energy and minerals, far less attention is paid to protein metabolism and protein requirements in horses. Particularly in the exercising horse, it is assumed that protein can be neglected if the feeding intensity increases in proportion to increased energy requirements. But there are some aspects which require more information, for example the prececal digestibility of protein and amino acids, the role of amino acids in exercising horses, and the impact of protein on performance.

1. Basic figures on protein metabolism used in deriving the system for protein requirements

The endogenous losses of nitrogen average at about 380 mg/kg metabolic body weight ($BW^{0.75}$). This figure is based on the results of various trials assessing endogenous fecal losses. Fecal nitrogen losses are dependent on nitrogen and dry matter intake. The best fitting equation is: fecal nitrogen losses (mg/kg $BW^{0.75}$ x day^{-1}) = $-234 + 2.56z + 0.2x + 10.4f - 0.08f^2$ (z = dry matter intake, g/kg $BW^{0.75}$ x day^{-1}; x = nitrogen intake, mg/kg $BW^{0.75}$ x day^{-1}; f = crude fiber, % of dry matter). Assuming an average crude fiber content of 20% in the ration, endogenous fecal losses will be 180 mg/kg $BW^{0.75}$ x day^{-1}.

Renal nitrogen excretion is in linear proportion to nitrogen intake (renal nitrogen excretion = 135 + 0.74 digestible nitrogen intake; excretion and intake in mg/kg $BW^{0.75}$ x d^{-1}). Endogenous renal losses are estimated at approximately 140 mg/kg $BW^{0.75}$.

For a factorial approach to protein requirements, data on cutaneous nitrogen losses should be considered, although they are generally low in the various species. It is dependent on hair growth and cell desquamation, and is assumed to be about 35 mg nitrogen/kg $BW^{0.75}$ x day^{-1}.

The sum of endogenous nitrogen losses (Table 1) can be calculated by the described figures. However, the endogenous fecal losses represent a synthesis of protein and differ in that respect from endogenous renal nitrogen losses. Therefore a 60% utilization rate of digestible protein for endogenous fecal losses is used to derive the basal nitrogen of ~250 mg nitrogen/kg $BW^{0.75}$ x day^{-1}. The amount of nitrogen delivered by secretion in the prececal section of the gastro-intestinal tract (Table 2) reflects the use of apparently digested nitrogen for different processes independent of nitrogen intake. Based on experimental data from balance studies, the utilization of digestible nitrogen for nitrogen turnover under maintenance conditions is 66%. This means that the minimum requirement for digestible protein (DCP) is 250/0.66 x 6.25 = 2.4 g DCP/kg $BW^{0.75}$. As both protein quality and the proportion of prececally digested protein vary between different feeds, under practical conditions the recommended supply of digestible crude protein is established at 3 g/kg $BW^{0.75}$ x day^{-1}.

For circumstances differing from maintenance, protein requirements depend on the ensuing products.

Table 1. Inevitable endogenous nitrogen losses (Meyer, 1984).

	mg/kg $BW^{0.75}$ x d^{-1}	Utilization of digestible protein, %	Basal nitrogen
via feces	180	60	72
via urine	140	-	140
via skin	35	-	35
			~250

Table 2. Nitrogen secretion into the lumen (Meyer 1984).

	ml/kg BW x d^{-1}	Nitrogen mg/kg BW x d^{-1}
Saliva	120	~90
Gastric secretion	40 - 70	~20
Bile	40	~4
Pancreatic secretion	100 - 120	~66

1.1 Pregnancy

Fetal growth is defined by an equation dependent on the day of gestation. Since more than 80% of fetal growth occur after day 200 of gestation, the last 4 months of pregnancy are most relevant to protein requirements in pregnant mares. Protein concentration in the fetus increases from approximately 100 up to 171 g crude protein/kg of fetal weight. The utilization of digestible crude protein for accretion in fetal tissues is assumed to be 50%. The percentages of energy and protein accretion are presented in Table 3. Base data used for digestible protein requirement during pregnancy are: digestible crude protein g/day = 0.06055 x a x $BW^{0.75}$ (a = protein accretion in % of total at birth; see Table 3).

Table 3. Energy and protein accretion in the fetus (GEH 1994).

Day of gestation	210		240		270		300		330
CP, g/kg BW_F	104		120		147		154		171
NE, MJ/kg BW_F	3.37		3.75		4.50		4.81		5.21
Accretion/month in % of total at birth		14		21.5		23		31	

F = Fetus

1.2 Milk synthesis

Milk yield and milk composition allow the calculation of protein requirements for lactation. Again, a utilization rate of 50% of digestible protein is assumed for milk synthesis.

Table 4. Dry matter, crude protein, and energy content of mare's milk per kg in correspondence with lactation stage (NRC 1989; GEH 1994).

Lactation stage in weeks	Milk quantity kg/kg $BW^{0.75}$ x d^{-1}	Dry matter g/kg	Crude protein g/kg	Energy[1] MJ/kg
1 - 4	0.14	107	27	2.44
5 - 8	0.17	105	22	2.32
9 - 21	0.12	100	18	2.12

[1] calculated with the following factors: protein 23.9, fat 39.5, lactose 17.5 kJ/g

1.3 Growth

To calculate protein requirements for growth, a model to estimate the growth rate and actual body weight of foals is essential. As shown in Figure 1, the body weight of foals (% of mature body weight) depends on current age and prospective body weight as an adult horse. The composition of the weight gain in the foal is calculated using equations for fat and protein (NRC, 1978; body fat % = 0.1388 x relative body weight + 1.11; body protein % = 0.22 x [100 - body fat]). The utilization of digestible protein for growth is 50% up to six months of age and 35% for older foals.

1.4 Work/Sweat

Nitrogen excretion via sweat is the only factor taken into consideration for calculating protein requirements in exercising horses. Sweat contains 1.25 g nitrogen/liter. Thus, although in hard working horses the additional protein requirement as a result of sweat production is low and is covered by the subsequently elevated feed intake.

Table 5 summarises the recommended daily energy and protein supply for horses of 400 and 600 kg BW.

2. Aspects calling for research

Although the formulation of a reasonable protein supply and the description of protein requirements is possible considering the different figures, there is still considerable need for further experimental work to elucidate certain aspects of protein requirements in horses.

The prececal digestibility of protein and amino acids should complete the basis, particularly for growing horses. Some amino acids have a remarkable influence on hormon systems, a rather important fact for mares (Sticker et al., 1999).

The protein intake in exercising hoses normally exceeds the protein requirement as derived regarding the previous data. There seems to be a benefit from rations low in protein. The acidogenic response during exercise was depressed after feeding less than 10% crude protein/kg total ration (Graham-Thiers et al., 1999). However, there still remains the question wether a supplemental intake of selected amino acids can improve horse´s performance. The oxydation of amino acids as a support of gluconeogenesis during exercise is examined in different species. The benefit of additional valine, isoleucine and leucine for exercising horses is still questionable. Obviously the carbon skeleton can be used for energy metabolism, but the changes in blood lactate do not indicate any relevant effect (Casini et al., 2000; Stefanon et al., 2000). The concentrations

Table 5. Recommendation for digestible energy (DE) and digestible crude protein (DCP) in horses (GEH, 1994).

Performance		BW, kg	DE, MJ/day	DCP, g/day
Maintenance		400	53.6	268
		600	32.6	318
Exercise, moderate		400	67-81	335-405
		600	91-109	455-545
Pregnancy,	9th - 11th month	400	70	420
		600	96	575
	11th month	400	74	420
		600	101	640
Lactation,	3rd month	400	105	875
		600	142	1185
Growth,	7th - 12th month	400[1]	57	475
		600[1]	74	610
	13th - 18th month	400[1]	59	400
		600[1]	77	560

[1] prospective weight at maturity

of ammonia in blood - the „byproduct" of amino acid oxydation - increase after feeding additional amino acids and in consequence the damand for urea synthesis and renal excretion is elevated.

The addition of of ß-alanine und L-histidine to the ration increased the concentration of carnosine in the equine muscle (Dunnett und Harris, 1999). Carnosine is an essential intracellular puffer and there a higher puffer capacity possibly can prevent critical changes in incellular pH. But ß-alanine utilisation can result in a taurine depletion of muscle and the muscle do not tolerance a big change in taurine. That needs to be investigated to have doubtless arguments for the use of those amnio acids in exercising horses.

The functions of branched chain amino acids and their role in central fatigue are also still unclear. To date it seems that serotonine is not involved in exercise-related response. If that is true, then tryptophan can be neglected in exercising horses. But experiments with supplemental Tryptophan yielded conflicting results (Farris et al., 1998; Vervuert et al., 2003). Therefore, the effect of tryptophan on the formation of neurotransmitters needs to be clarified in horses.

References

Casini, L., Gatta, D. Magni, L. and Colombani, B., 2000. Effect of prolonged branched-chain amino acid supplementation on metabolic response to anaerobic exercise in Standardbreds. J. Equine Vet. Sci. 20: 120-123.

Dunnett, M. and Harris, R.C., 1999. Influence of oral ß-alanine and L-histidine supplementation on the carnosine content of the gluteus medius. Equine Vet. J. Suppl. 30: 499-504.

Farris, J.W., Hinchcliff, K.W., McKeever, K.H., Lamb, D.R. and Thompson, D.L., 1998. Effect of tryptophan and of glucose on exercise capacity of horses. J. Appl. Physiol. 85: 807-816.

Gesellschaft Für Ernährungsphysiologie (GEH), 1994. Empfehlungen zur Energie und Nährstoffversorgung der Pferde. DLG-Verlag Frankfut/Main, ISBN 3-7690-0517-1 („Committee for requirement formulations of the German Society of Nutritional Physiology: Recommendations for the energy and nutrient supply for horses").

Graham-Thiers, P.M., Kronfeld, D.S. and Kline, K.A., 1999. Dietary protein influence acid-base responses to repeated sprints. Equine Vet. J. Suppl. 30: 463-467.

Meyer, H., 1984. Intestinaler N-Stoffwechsel, endogener N-Verlust und N-Bedarf ausgewachsener Pferde. Übersichten Tierernährung 12: 251-271.

National Research Council (NRC), 1978. Nutrient requirements of horses. 4th edition, National Academic Press, Washington D. C.

National Research Council (NRC), 1989. Nutrient requirements of horses. 5th edition, National Academic Press, Washington D. C.

Stefanon, B., Bettini, C. and Guggia, P., 2000. Administration of branched-chain amino acids to Standardbred horses in training. J. Equine Vet. Sci. 20: 115-119.

Vervuert, I., Coenen, M., Watermülder, E. and Zamhöfer, J., 2003. Effect of Tryptophan Supplementation on metabolic responses to exercise in horses. Equine Nutrition and Physiology Society, East Lansing, Michigan, 18: 287-288.

Protein requirements of horses for maintenance and work

Gary D. Potter

Equine Sciences, Department of Animal Science, Texas A&M University, College Station, Texas 77843

1. Flow of protein through the equine digestive tract

The following scheme, which describes the flow of feed protein through the equine digestive system is well established:

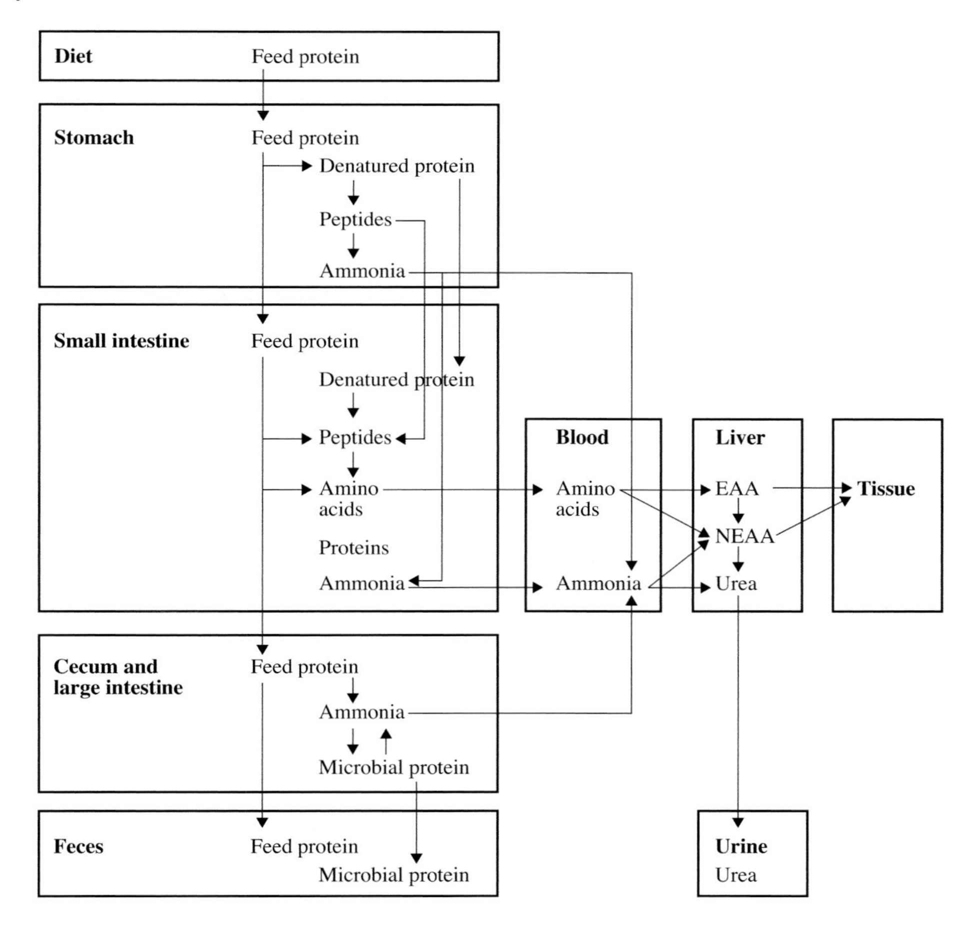

It is clear from this scheme that horses depend on a dietary source of essential amino acids (EAA) for synthesis of proteins in the tissues, and microbial protein synthesized in the cecum and large intestine is not a significant source of EAA for synthesis of protein in the tissues. It is well documented in the literature that young growing horses and lactating mares require a dietary source of EAA for maximal growth and milk production. Further, horses at maintenance can use ammonia generated from fermentation in the large intestine only to meet the nonessential amino acid (NEAA) requirement, thus, sparing the EAA supply from the diet (NRC, 1989). Thus, the protein requirements of horses, much like that of other nonruminants are actually amino acid requirements.

While the total-tract digestibility of nitrogen in a wide variety of feedstuffs is within a rather narrow range (typically 60-75%), not all feed proteins are not digested totally in the small intestine. Thus, the central question as to how to define protein requirements for horses depends entirely upon knowledge of the extent to which feed protein is digested in the small intestine, yielding both EAA and NEAA, or fermented in the cecum and large intestine, yielding ammonia. Simply stating the protein requirement in terms of digestible protein, when digestibility is calculated as the difference between intake and fecal excretion will not ensure that the horses' EAA requirements are met, even if some predicted digestible protein requirement is met. Thus, NRC (1989) gives only daily crude protein requirements, with reference to the importance of protein quality, because expression of daily requirements in terms of digestible protein can be extremely misleading-depending entirely on the location in the GI tract in which given feed proteins are digested.

2. Digestibility of feed proteins in different segments of the equine digestive tract

Development of a surgical technique to cannulate the distal small intestine (Peloso et al., 1994) has facilitated the study of digestion in different segments of the equine digestive tract. A major finding using that model was that passage of feed residues through the stomach and small intestine of the equine is comparatively fast (Nyberg et al., 1995). Mean residence time in the small intestine was found to be near 1.5 hours, which compares to 18-24 hours in the large intestine (Argenzio et al., 1974).

It is well known that the protein in forages is encapsulated in the plant cell, which is surrounded by cellulose and other structural fibers. Since there is no mammalian cellulase, and there is very little fermentation of forages in the stomach of the horse, a major question has been related to the extent to which forages can supply EAA for horses. Working with forages of varying quality, Gibbs et al. (1988) found that while the true digestibility of forage proteins was near 100%, the fraction of totally digestible protein that was digested in the small intestine of equines ranged from 2-29% (Table 1). The true digestibility of forage proteins in the equine small intestine was 37% compared to 96% in the large intestine, and plasma amino acid concentrations were elevated following consumption of only the higher quality forage. Farley (1995) found similar results in a subsequent study (figures 1, 2 and 3). While true digestibility of forage protein over the total tract was 90%, and that in the large intestine was 78%, true digestibility of forage protein in the small intestine was only 40%.

Clearly, these data indicate that the major site of forage protein digestion is in the large intestine of the equine, which results in production of ammonia rather than absorption of amino acids. Then, for forages to be a significant source of amino acids for horses, the forage must be of very high quality because the amino acids absorbed from the small intestine are apparently from only those proteins released by mastication of very immature, turgid material. It is important to note that in both studies, the true digestibility of forage proteins over the total tract and in the large intestine of equines is very high-90-100%. Thus, the fermentive action in the large intestine has a masking effect on digestion in the small intestine such that the total digestible protein in either low or high quality forages, as a fraction of the total protein, can appear similar. Therefore, it is futile to estimate the comparative usable protein in forages by measuring digestion at the end of the digestive tract. Similarly, it is difficult to assess the protein requirements of forage fed horses in terms of total digestible protein. Clearly, more research is needed to define regression equations

Table 1. Digestion of forage protein in different segments of the equine digestive tract (Gibbs et al., 1988).

	Bermuda grass	Low Alfalfa	High Alfalfa
N intake, mg/kg/meal	175[1]	221[2]	264[3]
N digested, mg/kg/meal			
Total tract	99[1]	146[2]	196[3]
Small intestine	17[1]	3[1]	56[2]
% of total	17.2	2.1	28.6
Large intestine	83[1]	143[2]	140[2]
% of total	83.8	97.9	71.4

[1,2,3] Means not sharing superscript are different (P<.05)

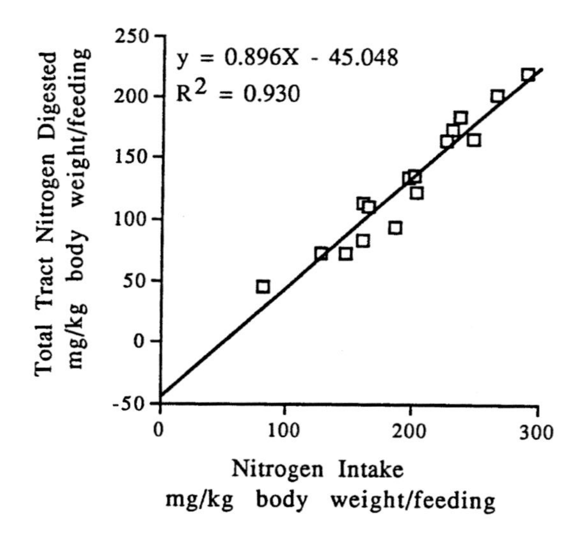

Figure 1. Forage nitrogen digestion in the total digestive tract of ponies (from Farley, 1995).

to predict the upper vs. lower tract digestion of forages as a function of nitrogen concentration, true protein concentration, NDF or other factors.

In contrast to findings in the all-forage fed horses, Farley et al. (1995) and Gibbs et al. (1996) found that digestion of cereal and oil-seed proteins was primarily in the small intestine of equines. As seen in Table 2, the portion of the digestible protein that was digested in the small intestine ranged from 50-95%. As seen in figures 4-6, true digestibility of soybean meal protein over the total tract was 96%, and that in the large intestine was 90%. Further, true digestibility of soybean meal protein in the small intestine was 72%. Even though cereal and oil-seen proteins were digested more extensively in the small intestine that the forage protein, as was the case for forage protein, any protein escaping digestion in the small intestine was almost totally fermented in the large intestine. Therefore, as stated earlier, measuring the digestibility of protein at the end of the equine digestive tract is almost meaningless to define the useable protein concentration in feeds. Thus, estimating protein requirements of horses in terms of digestible protein is potentially erroneous when nothing is known about the portion of protein in the diet that is digested in the

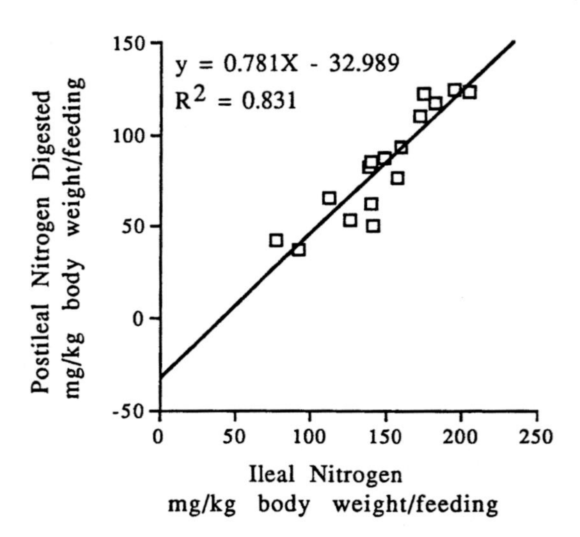

Figure 2. Forage nitrogen digestion in the large intestine of ponies (from Farley, 1995).

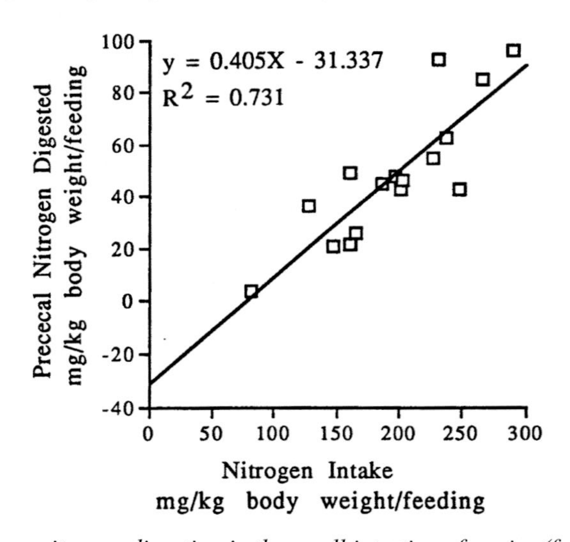

Figure 3. Forage nitrogen digestion in the small intestine of ponies (from Farley, 1995).

small intestine vs. the large intestine. More research is needed to define the upper tract digestibility of cereal and oil-seed proteins in horses and the effects of botanical source of protein, feed intake, feed processing, etc.

2.1 Capacity of the small intestine

Comparison of digestion of different feed proteins in the small intestine is shown in figure 7. From these data it appears that the capacity of the small intestine to digest protein (approximately 80 mg N/kgBW/meal) was reached in SBM-fed ponies at nitrogen intake of approximately 125 mg/kgBW/meal. Conversely, in forage fed ponies, it required nitrogen intake of approximately 300 mg/kgBW/meal to reach that same amount of small intestinal protein digestion. Thus, if one

Table 2. Digestion of supplemental cereal and oil-seed proteins in different segments of the equine digestive tract (Gibbs et al., 1996).

	Corn	Oats	Sorghum grain	SBM	CSM	Mean
N intake, mg/kg/meal	72	108	72	87	75	
N digested, mg/kg/meal						
Total tract	70	96	67	80	64	
Sm. Intest.	35	58	50	45	61	
% of total	50.0	60.4	74.6	56.2	95.3	67.3
Lrg. Intest.	35	38	17	35	3	
% of total	50.0	39.6	25.4	43.8	4.7	32.7

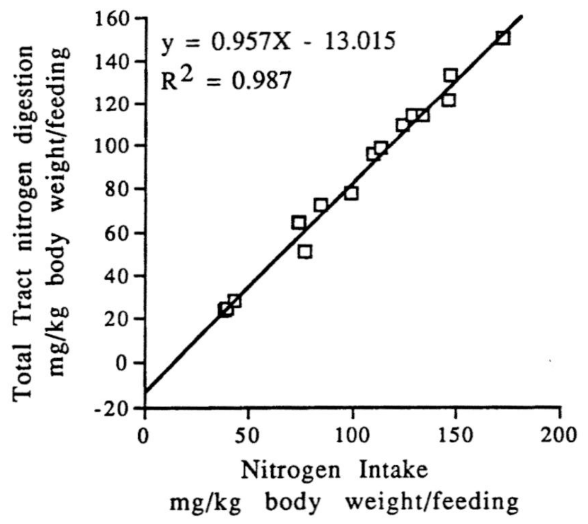

Figure 4. Digestion of soybean meal protein in the total tract of ponies (from Farley et al., 1995).

uses the maximal small intestinal protein digestion as a comparative estimate of the protein requirement, and assuming typical energy densities of concentrate and forage feeds, the protein concentration in forage feeds must be much higher than that in concentrate feeds to meet the horse's protein (amino acids) requirements. When high-protein forages are used to meet amino acid requirements of horses, excretions of nitrogen in both the feces and urine are very high. Excessive ammonia production in the large intestine may be harmful to horses, and it is surely environmentally challenging.

2.2 The NRC (1989) approach

Daily protein requirements of horses as recommended by NRC (1989) are in terms of crude protein, with reference to the importance of amino acid balance in the dietary protein. At the time of writing that publication, there were insufficient data in the literature to make recommendations beyond a daily requirement for dietary crude protein and a general discussion of the importance of amino acid balance in the dietary protein. Unlike the situation for energy, trying to account for protein lost in feces and using digestible protein to express the daily protein requirement was futile

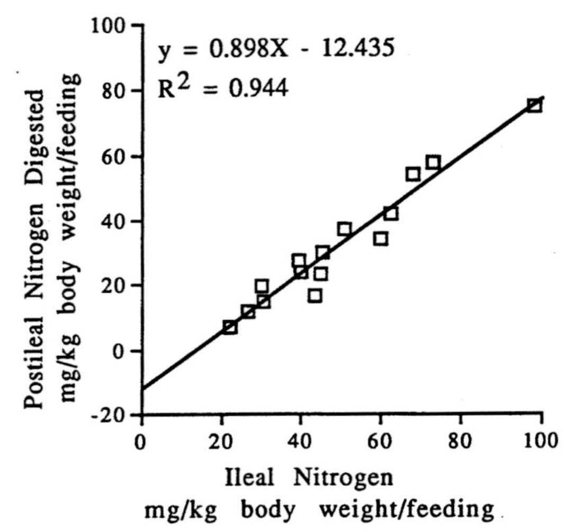

Figure 5. Digestion of soybean meal protein in the large intestine of ponies (from Farley et al., 1995).

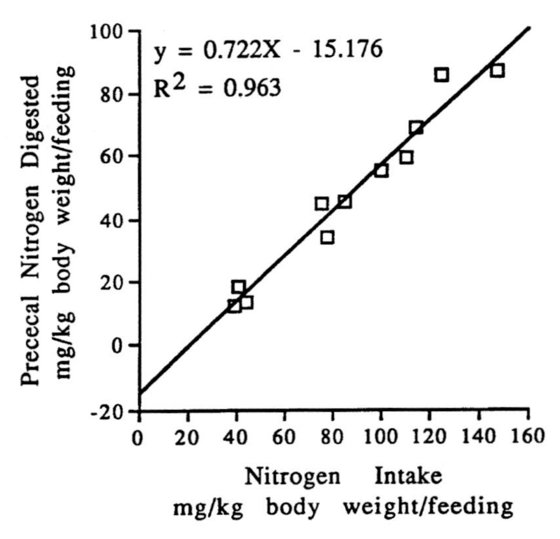

Figure 6. Digestion of soybean meal protein in the small intestine of ponies (from Farley et al., 1995).

at that time because there were too few data in the literature defining the digestion of protein in the small intestine vs. the large intestine in the horse.

2.3 The maintenance requirement

The NRC (1989) estimated the maintenance requirement of mature horses from research using nitrogen depletion/repletion techniques and nitrogen balance experiments (see references in NRC, 1989. Total tract digestible protein was used as the reference point, because the site of protein digestion in the mature horse at maintenance is less important than in other horses with higher protein requirements. That is because mature horses can utilize some of the nitrogen absorbed as

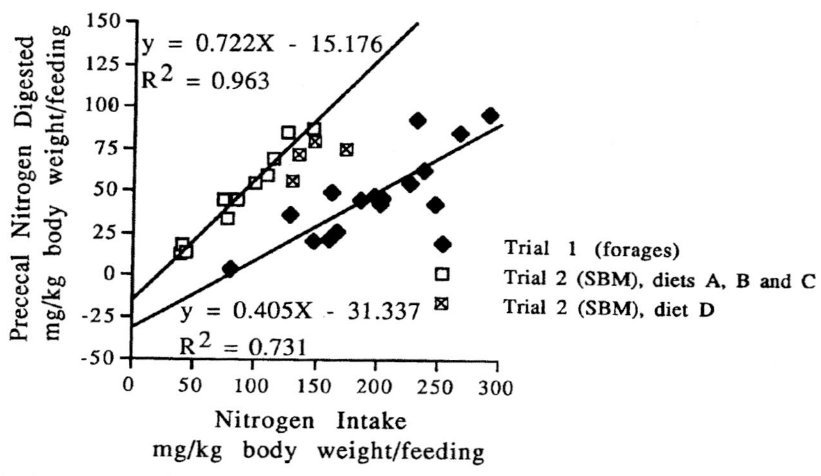

Figure 7. Comparative digestion of forage and SBM nitrogen in the small intestine of ponies (from Farley, 1995).

ammonia from the hindgut for synthesis of nonessential amino acids in the liver. Further, since protein requirements are related to energy requirements, the protein requirement for maintenance was calculated as 40 gm crude protein/Mcal DE. That protein/calorie ratio was then applied to energy requirements of horses of various sizes and stages of production to estimate the maintenance requirement for crude protein. In all cases, NRC (1989) recommended that the dietary protein for horses, even at maintenance should contain 3.5% lysine. This was done to ensure some degree of focus on the importance of protein quality in formulating diets for horses.

2.4 The protein requirement for work

Freeman et al. (1988) found that nitrogen retention in exercising horses increased as workload increased, but it was not necessary to increase the protein density in the diet to meet the extra requirements for muscular hypertrophy and nitrogen lost in sweat (figure 8). When a diet of

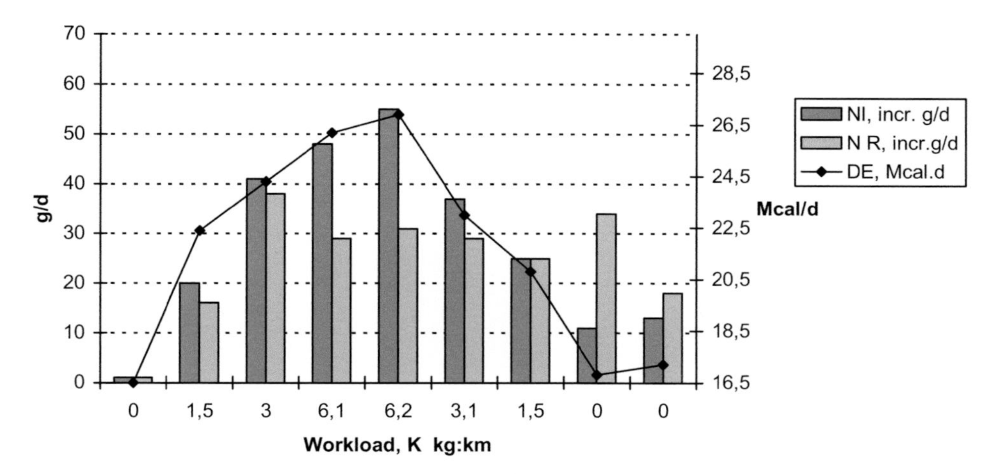

Figure 8. Nitrogen retention in working horses (from Freeman et al., 1988).

constant protein:calorie ratio was fed to meet DE requirements, daily nitrogen intake increased from 180 to 294 mg/kg BW. Daily nitrogen absorption increased from 124 mg/kg BW to 208 mg/kg BW, and nitrogen retention increased from 23 to 83 mg/kg BW. An increase in daily nitrogen intake of 114 mg/kg BW resulted in increased daily nitrogen absorption of 84 mg/kg BW and daily nitrogen retention of only 60 mg/kg BW. Calculating from the data of Freeman et al. (1988), it is possible that the protein requirement of those exercising horses was approximately 32 g CP/Mcal DE.

Thus, these data and others led the NRC (1989) to conclude that when a diet containing sufficient protein to meet the maintenance requirement (40 g CP/Mcal DE) is fed to meet the DE requirement, the diet will supply sufficient protein to meet any increased protein requirements due to work. As a practical matter, and to provide recommendations useable in the feed and horse industry, protein requirements in the NRC (1989) tables were computed from the ratio of 40 gm CP/Mcal DE. Thus, the data in Tables 5-1, A-G, of NRC (1989) which reflect daily protein requirements for working horses are likely higher than the actual daily protein requirement. Conversely, recommended dietary protein density as shown in Tables 5-2, A-B, of NRC (1989) indicate that any increase in the required protein density in the diet of working horses is very small.

References

Argenzio, R.A, Lowe, J.E. Pickard, D.W. and Stevens, C.E., 1974. Digesta passage and water exchange in the equine large intestine. Am. J. Physiol. 226: 1035.

Farley, E.B., 1995. Digestion of protein in the equine small and large intestine. M.S. Thesis. Texas A&M University Library. College Station, TX., USA.

Farley, E.B., Potter, G.D. Gibbs, P.G. Schumacher, J.and Murray-Gerzik, M., 1995. Digestion of soybean meal protein in the equine small and large intestine at varying levels of intake. J. Equine Vet. Sci. 15(9): 391.

Freeman, D.W., Potter, G.D. Schelling, G.T. and Kreider, J.L., 1988. Nitrogen metabolism in mature horses at varying levels of work. J. Anim. Sci. 66: 407.

Gibbs, P.G., Potter, G.D. Schelling, G.T. Kreider, J.L. and Boyd, C.L., 1988. Digestion of hay protein in different segments of the equine digestive tract. J. Anim. Sci. 66: 400.

Gibbs, P.G., Potter, G.D. Schelling, G.T. Kreider, J.L. and Boyd, C.L., 1996. The significance of small vs. large intestinal digestion of cereal grain and oilseed protein in the equine. J. Equine Vet. Sci. 162(2): 60.

National Research Council, 1989. Nutrient Requirements of Horses. 5th rev. ed. Washington, D.C.:National Academy Press.

Peloso, J.G., Schumacher, J. McClure, S.R. Crabill, M.R. Hanselka, D.V. Householder, D.D. and Potter, G.D., 1994. Technique for long-term ileal cannulation in ponies. Can. J. Vet. Res. 58: 181.

Nyberg, M.A., Potter, G.D. Gibbs, P.G. Schumacher, J. Murray-Gerzik, M. Bombarda, A. and Swinney, D.L., 1995. Flow rate through the equine small intestine determined with soluble and insoluble indicators. Proc. 14th Equine Nutr. Phys. Symp. p. 36.

Evaluating the protein requirements of performance horses: A comparison of practical application of different systems

Dag Austbø

Department of Animal Science, Agricultural University of Norway

The protein requirements of horses are expressed in different terms by different systems, as crude protein (CP), apparent digestible crude protein (DCP) or horse digestible crude protein (MADC). The protein requirement increases with increasing work load (exercise), and in all systems the protein:energy ratio is about the same for work as for maintenance.

1. Calculation of protein requirements

According to the USA system (NRC, 1989), protein requirements for maintenance and work are calculated as 40 g of CP per Mcal of digestible energy (DE). When arriving at this value, a daily requirement of 0.60 g DCP per kg BW was used. For a 500 kg horse, this is equivalent to 2.8 g of DCP/kg $BW^{0.75}$. A protein digestibility of 46% is used and the CP requirement is calculated to be 1.3 g/kg BW/day (6.1 g/kg $BW^{0.75}$). This low value for digestibility is related to a maintenance ration mainly consisting of roughage of moderate quality. The system does not take into account the increased use of concentrates in rations for exercised horses.

In Germany protein requirements for maintenance and work are calculated as 3 grams DCP/$BW^{0.75}$, or as 5 grams DCP per MJ DE (DLG, 1992). The same system (3 grams DCP/ $BW^{0.75}$)) is used in Holland (CVB, 1996).

In France a new protein evaluation system has been developed (Martin-Rosset, 2000). In this system the protein value of feedstuffs for horses is expressed as the sum of feed and microbial amino acids absorbed in the small and large intestine and referred to as Horse Digestible Crude Protein (MADC). The system is based on the calculation of DCP requirements for maintenance, 2.4 g DCP/kg$BW^{0.75}$. In comparison with MADC values, DCP overestimates the protein value of forages by 10 - 30%. As a result, the requirements for MADC for maintenance is increased to 2.8g/kg $BW^{0.75}$ (74g MADC/UFC). For exercise the requirement is 65-70 g MADC/UFC. The MADC content of the main groups of forages is calculated by multiplying their DCP content using a factor K. K=0.9 for green forages, 0.85 for hay and dehydrated forages, 0.7 for good quality grass silages. For concentrates the K is 1.0 (no correction).

2. Comparison of the different systems

To compare requirements for protein according to the different systems, protein is expressed as DCP in all systems. When calculating DCP from CP a digestibility of 46% is used, as well as digestibilities calculated using different roughage:concentrate ratios as exercise is increased. When calculating DCP from MADC the K-values are used (Table 1.)

For Germany and Holland the requirements for DCP are identical as in both countries the basis for calculation is the same (3 grams of DCP/kg $BW^{0.75}$ for maintenance, and the same protein:energy ratio for exercise).

The NRC-system uses CP, but the values for maintenance and exercise are based on DCP using 0.6 g DCP/kg BW for maintenance and the same protein:energy ratio for exercise.

Table 1. Protein requirements of performance horses (500 kg BW) according to different systems.

System	Exercise				
	Maint.	1.25*Maint.	1.5*Maint.	1.75*Maint.	2.0*Maint.
NRC, CP	656	820	984	1148	1312
NRC, DCP[1]	302	377	453	528	604
DCP[2]	302	500	615	751	899
NL Mare, DCP	317	397	476	555	634
NL Stallion, DCP	349	436	523	611	698
Germany, DCP	318	397	476	556	635
France, MADC	295	365	435	505	575
France, DCP[3]	347	415	483	555	618
France, DCP[4]	254	317	381	444	508

[1] DCP calculated using digestibility of 46%

[2] DCP calculated using digestibilities of 46 - 61 - 62.5 - 65 - 68.5%

[3] DCP calculated using K-values 0.85 - 0.88 - 0.9 - 0.91 - 0.93

[4] DCP calculated using 2.4 g DCP*$BW^{0.75}$ * Exercise intensity

A digestibility of 46% is used independent of ration (roughage:concentrate). When calculating from CP to DCP using a digestibility of 46%, the values correspond quite well with the German and Dutch figures. If, however, actual digestibilities are being used, the calculated DCP requirements will be higher.

In France the maintenance requirement for DCP was set to 2.4 g/kg $BW^{0.75}$. When MADC is used, the value is 2.8 g MADC/kg $BW^{0.75}$. Since the requirements were increased in the MADC system, recalculating to DCP gives higher values compared to the original 2.4 g/kg $BW^{0.75}$.

Examples of how the requirement for DCP can be calculated according to the different systems are shown in table 1. The basis for calculating maintenance protein requirements is 2.8-3.0 grams of DCP/kg $BW^{0.75}$, except for the French system (3.3 g DCP/kg $BW^{0.75}$).

3. Amino acids

Lysine and possibly threonine is the most limiting amino acids for horses. In general, the amino acid requirements of adult horses at maintenance and work will be met under normal feeding conditions. The NRC system gives guidelines for lysine requirements for adult horses at maintenance and work as 0.035*g of CP/day.

References

CVB, 1996. Documentatierrapport nr 15. Het definitieve VEP-en VREp-systeem, Central Veevoederbureau, Lelystad.

DLG, 1992. Empfehlungen zur Energie-und Nährstoffversorgung der Pferde, DLG-Verlag, Frankfurt/Main

NRC, 1989. Nutrient Requirements of Horses, 5th ed. revised, National Academy of Sciences, Washington DC.

Martin-Rosset, W., 2000. Feeding Standards for Energy and Protein for Horses in France, Advances in Equine Nutrition ll, Kentucky Equine Research Inc., Versailles, Kentucky, USA, 245-303.

Printed in the United States
by Baker & Taylor Publisher Services